Women and the Liberating

Journey of Aging

Women and the Liberating Journey of Aging

Awakening fire in the heart

Marilyn Loy Every, DMin

Book Cover Design: Trista Baldwin
Editor: Sue Kehoe
Assistant Editor: Nina Shoroplova
Production Editor: Jennifer Kaleta
Typeset: Greg Salisbury

Dedication

♥

For my mother
Grace Nelsen Loy
(1914-2006)

This book is dedicated to you
and to your infinite light
that continues to shine
through the lives
of those you dearly love.

In Women and the Liberating Journey of Aging, *Dr. Loy Every challenges the limitations culturally imposed upon the fully mature Western woman. She offers a wise, integrated holistic vision— Sagessence—that will open your eyes to your beauty and infuse your heart with hope. A book brimming with wisdom and insight...*

Rev. Dr. Lauren Artress
Author, *Walking a Sacred Path* and
The Sacred Path Companion

Acknowledgements

♥

I am deeply grateful to have amazing, inspiring, and transforming influences in my life. All are reflected throughout the entire writing of this book, as well as the outcome. The message of *Women and the Liberating Journey of Aging—Awakening fire in the heart* simply would not be published without the support of so many talented, competent, gifted, and beloved people who have come into my life. I am a better person because of each of these women and men. My heart is filled with great love and gratitude for the journey that has led me to this moment in time. I humbly hold each of you with the spirit of *Namaste*.

With gratitude,

Love and deep appreciation, I acknowledge my mother, Grace, and grandmother, Sophia. I am grateful for your choices that gave me life. Without your lives and legacies, questions which were foundational for *Women and the Liberating Journey of Aging—Awakening fire in the heart* would have never been asked. I honor you in every word of this book. As you continue to live through me, together we tell our stories as well as those of other women. My journey reflects the legacy of your spirits.

With gratitude,

I acknowledge the wise women whose lives and voices accompanied me through every page and chapter of this book. Thank you especially to Ruth, "Hedda," Lily, Elene, Edith, Nancy, Maria, Lavina, Mary, and Louise. Your stories are treasures. Your truths offer women courageous inspiration, and your wisdom gives us valuable guidance.

With gratitude,
I acknowledge Jennifer, Kristen, Nina, and Annie for your inspiring ideas, choices, and ways of living authentic legacies. I see you standing as exemplars for our younger generation of women. Your stories enrich my life, and your brilliant lights shine forth to light the way for many others.

With gratitude,
I acknowledge the sacred circles of wise women with whom I share my life. Each of you has helped to shape the texture of my writing simply by your presence in my life. My dedication to re-envisioning women in the second half of life has been viewed through a lens of rich wisdom each of you shares. Your belief in my vision of *Sagessence* has been fuel for the fire in my heart.

With gratitude,
I acknowledge and honor Rev. Dr. Lauren Artress, Dr. Kathleen Fischer, Dr. Joan Borysenko, and Dr. Jean Houston, innovative "sage leaders," torchbearers for the good of women, our communities, and the Earth. Each of you has and continues to gift the world with priceless and wise gems. You are cherished mentors and esteemed women who have piloted my voice throughout my writing, poetry, and ministry in the world.

With gratitude,
I acknowledge and bow with a spirit of reverence to the spiritual teachers who have touched my life deeply,

and who have high regard for women and their sacred journeys. Your voices speak on the pages of this book. I give particular heartfelt thanks to the ministries of Matthew Fox—Episcopal priest and Christian theologian, the 14th Dalai Lama—Tibetan monk, and 15th century Christian mystics—Hildegard von Bingen and Meister Eckhart.

With gratitude,

I acknowledge Dr. John Hanagan. As my doctoral mentor, you provided encouragement and valued guidance for my musings and queries relative to re-envisioning aging in our culture. You offered a masculine balance to our dialogue as we explored feminine aspects of aging. Sincere appreciation is extended to my content specialist and spiritual advisor, Dr. Alexandra Kovats. You imparted great depths of female wisdom while relentlessly and lovingly believing in and supporting my vision. And, thank you to Jennifer Hager, my organizational editor; your keen and curious expertise prompted me toward new explorations over and again.

With gratitude,

I acknowledge Julie Salisbury, President and CEO of Influence Publishing, who welcomed my vision, believed in my mission, and supported my endeavor in every step of bringing this message to women. Thank you to each person on her team, particularly Sue Kehoe, my manuscript editor, whose insight and expertise affected the amazing outcome. I consider you all the "Red Tent" mid-wives for *Women and the Liberating Journey of Aging—Awakening fire in the heart.*

With gratitude,

And enduring love, I acknowledge the support and love of my beloved family. As your love surrounds me, indeed, I am buoyed by a sacred wind beneath my wings. Together we continue to weave a fabulous tapestry of legacy keeping in mind our own unique abilities to live for higher good—for our generations, and beyond. Simply, it is for you, my children and grandchildren, I aspire to be a worthy sage as I illuminate my own *Sagessence* into the world.

Contents

Foreword

♥

As someone who has worked in human development in 109 countries, I can attest to the truth of this book, *Women and the Liberating Journey of Aging—Awakening fire in the heart*. All over the world and with few exceptions, we find that it is women "of a certain age"—seasoned women—who are taking the initiative across a wide spectrum of personal and social change. Having seen their children grown, and other children they have nurtured to maturity, they seem less fearful of the personal consequences of taking risks, creating and following through on needed communal projects—disciplining, inspiring, teaching, and making things happen! Post-menopausal zest is a living fact and its consequences may well be the saving of the human race and the betterment of the planet. Equally important, Dr. Marilyn Loy Every, the author of this elegant work, shows how *Sagessence* is leading to the obsolescence of "ageism." Move forward through each page of her message to women and dare to be transformed by espousing the emerging archetype of the sage.

Jean Houston, PhD
Author of twenty-eight books on human and social development
Consultant to the United Nations Development Program

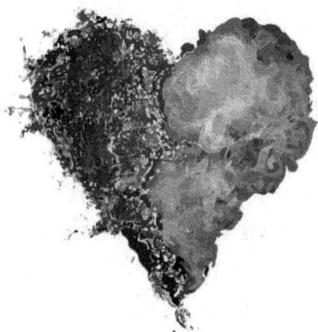

Vision of Sagessence

I come to you
to reveal a vision that
tumbles inside, condensed,
contained, living rib to rib.
Where shall be a next step?
Is it earth in our tread?
Or, an imprint yet to recede
into fresh, new, fertile soil?

Shall we rest in the settled dust
of culture's past knowing?
Or, lift our feet up
anticipating a daring turn?
Shall we tiptoe to the edge
of society's comfort and gaze,
or collapse into arms
of Wisdom's sacred abyss?

Turning an ear to muffled,
distant heart sounds, implore,
"Please foretell the story that
the Ancient Ones prophesied."
Then comes a deep whisper
rising through dense history,
You are a sage; and
I bid your holy consecration.

O fervent sages—
Draw from your wells,
illuminate your Sagessence,

shine forth your sacred story.
Enliven the cosmic story!
The breath of god waits
to bless what only you can live . . .
yes, wisdom only you can give.

Be it, too, your vivid vision,
with your sacred flame aglow . . .
walking on, hands high,
and freedom
breathing in your soul,
assured
the breath of god awaits . . .
your Sagessence story.[1]

Introduction

The Alchemy

♥

Grace wanted to be called "Grace." My mother didn't want to be called "Mrs.," although she had been married sixty-six years, and was crazy in love with my father. She wanted her own identity. One way was not to be called "dear," "honey," or "Mrs." After years of failing health, Grace died when she was ninety-two years old. Her last six months of life were very difficult. I flew from Seattle to the Midwest ten times in those months, each time an urgent departure due to yet another critical situation. She fell and broke her hip that February. She had fallen many times in later years, but this time she was hospitalized. Amazingly, it was the first time she had been a patient in a hospital since I was born.

Unfortunately, after that fatal fall, my mother then lived the rest of her life in a nursing home. Grace detested the fact that she could only take a bath every three days due to nursing care protocol. A daily bubble bath had been her treasured way of luxuriating self-care since the day she, my father, brothers, and I moved into a house with inside plumbing. She was also embarrassed, actually disgusted, that she needed to use a call light, and frustrated to wait and wait for a nurse's aide to find time to assist her to the bathroom. She was angry that a staff person came and grabbed the red walker my father bought for her—that pesky walker that had finally become her dear friend. The nurse's aide took it without Grace's permission for someone else to use. Generally, Grace was a good sport. She was a god-loving woman. She was kind-hearted, generous, polite, and proper. My mother worked hard to regain her strength in order to return home, and played by all the rules to get there.

My frail father diligently planted a plethora of flowers along the gravel driveway in front of the garage. He continued his farming skills of planting, fertilizing, and watering. He nursed all those flowers with tender care so they would be blooming when his beloved wife returned home. There was no question how happy she would be to see the black plastic barrels brimming over with so many blossoms. That August, Grace finally got to go home for an afternoon visit to see if she and Dad could manage her living there relative to her new level of physical care. I was told that, after the home assessment, she looked into my father's eyes and said, "You will never be able to take care of me here again." She died three days later.

On that night my mother passed, I received a call about 11:00 p.m. When the phone rang, I fumbled for it on the nightstand. I suddenly sensed the upcoming of nausea in the pit of my stomach. It had been two weeks since my father trumped my mother's wishes that she not be resuscitated. This time, her daughter knew her intentions. The voice at the other end of the conversation said Grace had been transported back to the hospital once again. I knew intuitively that she meant business this time and there was no time for me to be with her. My father later shared with me that she kept muttering, "Let's get going!" I am certain she was commanding the entourage of angels and guides that surrounded her that night.

I rolled over in bed, swung my feet to the floor, and swept my robe around my shoulders. I slowly gauged each step as I moved down the stairs in the dark. I flipped the light switch on in the kitchen to brew a cup of tea. Opening the cupboard door, I reached for the cup with "Love" inscribed in a big red heart. Pouring hot steaming water into the cup my mother always liked to use when she visited, I swamped a ginger teabag. Cradling the cup in my hands, I shuffled to my meditation room and lit a candle. In the silence of the night, I sat alone in my own darkness praying for her ease and comfort. Without hesitancy, my little dogs, Emy and Eli, took their watchful positions as tears began to stream down my face. Emy scooted up to the back of the chair cushion; Eli nestled next to me with his head compassionately resting in my lap. Time crawled by as I watched the mystery of candlelight shadows dancing on the walls.

I reflected on my mother's life, as I knew it, and wondered what I didn't know. She was the youngest child of a Danish family that settled in Custer County, Nebraska. They were farmers. She married my dad when she was twenty-six. That was considered an old age in 1939 for a woman to marry out there on the plains of the Midwest. As the youngest daughter, expectations were that my mother would not marry, but care for her parents throughout their lives. However, my mother managed to date my father in some fashion for four years. Not only had she stepped out-of-bounds of the family expectations, but she had also courted a younger man. My dad sent her a letter of proposal from Minnesota to Nebraska, and within two weeks, she married him. Needless to say, my grandfather was not happy with her decision. On her wedding day, my

♥

grandfather gave her $50 cash to cover her expenses when she got her wits about her and returned home.

Grace proved to be a good wife and partner. Her role was to be the grease in my dad's cogs as he worked hard at their livelihood of farming, ranching, and dairy. She made our family of five run as smoothly as she could, always trying to have what we needed in place and on time. She had two miscarriages before I was born which, she told me once, broke her heart. That was a silent sadness she tucked away in her otherwise busy rural life.

During a conversation I had with my mother when she was in her eighties, I asked how she thought her life would have been different. She said that she thought she would have married a minister, which would probably have been an acceptable marriage to her strictly religious father. We both laughed, yet I understood that idea really had been her dream as a young woman. My father was a far cry from a minister! He was the most fun-loving, mischievous prankster that I had ever known, and he was a bit irreverent when she allowed it. His sanctuary was nature although she managed to corral him into church every Sunday. I asked what she dreamed that she might have done in her life and didn't do. She said she always wanted to be a secretary, yet she had never "worked," comparing herself to women who had causes and careers other than being a housewife. (She mused about a revised title of "housewife" to "domestic engineer" that she wanted to report as her occupation to the Internal Revenue Service.) We had a long conversation about how she could still satisfy those dreams. She ingeniously decided to become a volunteer for the parish office at her church. She found her own "ministry" while working in the business office of that large parish.

❦

Curled up with a warm throw in the dark that night, I reminisced how different my mother's life was from her mother's life. Grandma Sophia was in a wheelchair for thirty years from rheumatoid arthritis that crippled her body to an inflexible stump. She essentially lived in two rooms of her house to limit her need to navigate. I remembered her shoe leather cut open to accommodate her gnarly toes; her hands were twisted to clumps in her lap. Grandma lived without the relief of pain management that is available with today's pharmaceuticals. However, she never complained, even when I frequently sat on her lap, which must have caused her great physical discomfort. She always sat quietly with a slight smile on her face in the quiet seclusion of my grandpa and grandma's huge old country farmhouse.

My mom, on the other hand, spent thirty years wrestling with a chronic lung condition that ultimately took her life. Yet, in her late eighties, she learned to turn a computer on, master email, and relentlessly barrage her senators with her political opinions. Admirably, she was committed to making calls from her bed in the nursing home to arrange volunteers for parish services and activities, even in her last weeks of life. She was devoted to her service.

Grace never ran for president other than for her club with the neighborhood ladies. She never wrote a book other than her diaries. My mother never climbed a mountain although she stood with me on snow-topped Hurricane Ridge without a coat, her arms waving in the air and brimming with a wonderful, huge smile. She traveled whenever she and my father could, and never met a stranger along her way.

It was 4:17 a.m. when I felt it in my body that my mother

had passed. The candle on the hearth flickered, like it was time to be snuffed out. I called the hospital one last time. Our Grace had died at 4:10 a.m. That early foggy morning, I grabbed a fleece jacket from the hall closet and stepped out on the front porch still wearing my pajamas. I breathed in deeply the welcomed cool, misty air, and started to walk down the street. Slight light of an impending dawn glazed the mountains across the Hood Canal that August morning.

I wondered, "Now that she is gone, who am I now?" Actually, I was a motherless daughter and the oldest woman in my family at fifty-six years of age. That's who I was. It was a quiet transition from daughter to oldest woman. It certainly wasn't as if I hadn't had time to consider my impending role. Yet I had no preparation. There were no manuals, guidelines, nor rituals. There was no gala occasion, ceremony, nor certificate of acknowledgement. What did it all mean? What was I to do, if anything? I didn't need acknowledgement, for certain. No other woman I knew had even talked about a moment like this. I needed discernment. Maybe I could ask Mom. Yet, snapping into reality, I remembered she was now gone.

Months passed, and in November following my mother's death, I met with my doctoral advisor, Dr. John Hanagan. We were discussing over lunch the subject matter of my dissertation. My intent was to explore possibilities of re-envisioning aging in a culture that reveres early life and considers elders with lessening regard during the passing of their years. I shared with him that it just so happened that in the middle of my process of discernment regarding the focus of my dissertation that my mother had passed away. Up close and personal, I had begun to grapple

♥

with picturing my role as eldest female in my *tribe*. The conventional matriarch model that was embedded in my female heritage did not fit my idea of family leadership. As I pondered the notion of *matriarch* and aging per se, I felt an inner urgency to visualize a different dynamic woman leadership model. I imagined a paradigm that was broader and had more potential to synergistically effect change. Dr. Hanagan challenged me to define what that leadership role might be for women, and encouraged me to define it as central to the dissertation.

I began reflecting on all of the older women I have had the privilege of working with in various capacities over the years. I have witnessed astonishing womanly strength, steadfast grit, and unfailing determination, as maturing women wrestled with ways to create the life they dreamed. I began to realize as I started my day each morning with a look in the bathroom mirror that I was gazing into the face of a woman who was also known for her grit, and was well on her way through her sixth decade.

I realized that every day of my workweek, I looked forward to encountering yet another woman who was over the age of fifty. I was fascinated as I watched and learned how women tend to become better with life! My curiosity was impetus to gain insight as I engaged in frank conversations with women about post-menopausal life. It became clear that our society needs us, and the wisdom of all our years. Ours is a unique wisdom that can only emerge from living the sacred journey of our amazing, unique life. I wondered, "Why does our culture ignore this?"

Actually, my desire to make a difference in the ways our culture responds to maturing women was sparked some fifteen years prior to the writing of the doctoral dissertation. I began consciously taking action for change while completing coursework for a graduate degree in counseling psychology. I worked primarily with older women as a grief and transition counselor. I marveled at the unique magnificence I witnessed in each woman as they encountered challenges and made efforts to transform their lives. Many courageously initiated new beginnings resulting from imposed or chosen personal change that in turn also effected variations in their relationships, families, and communities. Life changes also impacted decisions relative to continuing or discontinuing careers, as well as retirement plans. Of course, there were also end-of-life challenges that tossed usual life sideways and redefined ways of living, whether they were their own situations, or circumstances of people who impacted them.

It became apparent that what many maturing women actually longed for were richer relationships and deeper connections. They longed for dignity and to be treated with respect. Women hungered to increase self-actualization no matter what their situation presented. Many desired to deepen in consciousness and increase an outpouring of loving energy toward their families, and beyond. Most often, there were concerns about how to create a better quality of life. They understood that a by-product of satisfying such longings resulted in remarkable contributions to a more sustainable world. I recognized their amazing potential to create possibilities: to live influential legacies, and to wisely increase enrichment for their lives which in turn positively impacted people around them. Those women, as well as my mother and grandmother, were the women who actually were "midwives" for my commitment to explore greater liberty for women living in the second half of life.

❦

Furthermore, throughout a long-standing career in audiology, I provided hearing healthcare for a high percentage of patients over the age of fifty and upwards to centenarian patients. Regardless of a female patient's age, as a healthcare provider, I was absolutely committed to addressing individual needs and goals with respect, while honoring her dignity and integrating her own decision-making relative to care. I saw many family members attempt to speak for their mothers. Without including their mothers in the conversation, they boldly decided what care options would be chosen. It was always imperative to communicate empathically with genuine interest in the patients' topics of concern, whether it was concerns relative to communicating with family members, establishing care in a new community, or the timing of services in the midst of a terminal illness. Daily encounters like these afforded many opportunities to further examine my beliefs and values regarding aging.

As I continued to ponder how to create a positive shift in our culture regarding aging women, and to imagine a life-affirming leadership model, pressing questions came to mind. I wondered, "How can re-envisioning women's aging in the second phase of womanhood provide opportunities to enrich women's lives?" "How would it enrich my life?" "How would re-envisioning women's aging further my psychological, relational, social, and spiritual development, as well as benefit other women?"

It became clear to me that as women explore a reframing of maturity, we gain a new foundation to positively transform views and practices that have confined us. Certainly, to initiate change, we have a responsibility to confront typical cultural stances and do our diligent work to create liberating images, practices, and lifestyles. Of course, meaningful change begins within our own personal lives.

I am reminded of an elderly woman, Rachel, who came up to me following a seminar I facilitated, "Women, Wisdom, and the Power of Aging." Her eyes appeared sad as she asked, "How can I change the way my family sees me?" I suggested she might start by changing the way she saw herself. "Ahhh," she said, slowly nodding her head up and down. You see, we can't really change other people. However, we can certainly change ourselves by transforming our ideals and beliefs, and thereby our behaviors. When we challenge the views we have of ourselves, the way we live our lives, and the manner in which we view the world, we begin a new process of transformation.

Have you ever wondered how you can personally shift cultural views toward more positive and inspiring views of aging? How will you choose to live into the latter years of your life in meaningful ways? What exciting choices are you making to create a rich, fulfilling journey in the years to come? Metaphorically speaking, how can you awaken fire in your heart, and dance in the transforming heat of your one beautiful, incredible, maturing life until your last breath?

These are the questions that are the basis of *Women and the Liberating Journey of Aging—Awakening fire in the heart*. As you read the following chapters of this book, I encourage you to take time to read contemplatively, and take time to reflect on your own life with reverence. Explore the ideas, stories, and poetry from a vantage point that carries you deeper into your own heart of discernment, inspiration, and wisdom. May you recognize and hold dear

❤

your own illumination of wisdom-in-action shining forth into the world. Begin to imagine liberating possibilities arising from all of your life experiences. Accept that your life is fertile ground for further awakening liberating gifts yet to be revealed. Therefore, in honoring and celebrating the unfolding journey of maturing women, I invite you on this journey—*Women and the Liberating Journey of Aging.*

Marilyn Loy Every

Author, with fire in her heart

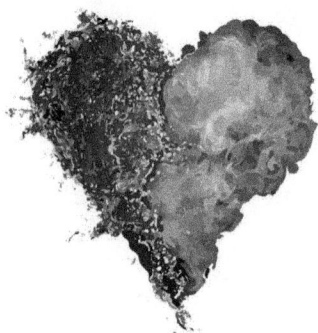

Chapter 1

The Sage Coming of Age

❤

Traditional and matriarchal societies have honored the older woman's power. Older women have been viewed as "wise women."[1] She has been known as midwife, herbalist, healer, and teacher. Using her insight and wisdom gained from years of experience, she becomes advisor, judge, and arbiter for her tribe and community. As crone, she is holy fury. She is a wellspring of resourceful knowledge and profound wisdom. The wise woman becomes leader of ceremonies, rituals, celebrations, and for every event from birth to death. Her intelligence, her logic of life balance, and sense of humor are at its peak in her elder years. Her vocation is that of furthering the well-being of the planet, and to the far-reaches of impacting the cosmos. The mature woman has learned to walk in the ways of beauty, poise, and spiritual power. This vision is compelling in its rich image of an older woman. However, in cultures where the elder woman is feared, rejected, dismissed, or not even acknowledged, these functions are denied her.

Cultural Views of Aging Women

Understanding cultural views of the aging process for women is crucial to ascertaining the challenges that women face as they age. Women encounter typical societal views of declining personal value and diminishing returns. Their aging has been associated with increasing vulnerability, uselessness, powerlessness, unattractiveness, and fragility. Other stereotypical inferences include diminished physical attractiveness and decreased sexual desirability. Unless we reframe our view of aging, we will continue to deprive our families, communities, and society of the full experiences that older women have to offer.

Numerous images have dictated how aging women have been viewed in our culture. For example, it is startling to read the definition of "crone" in *Webster's Dictionary*: "a withered, witchlike old woman."[2] One wonders how this authority could divert so diametrically from a bumper sticker I saw recently: "CRONE Creative Researcher of New Experiences."

Dr. Kathleen Fischer, forerunner for aging women and author of *Autumn Gospel*, states, "Older women, like old forests, are not highly valued by our society. The term itself has unpleasant connotations. Words like crone and hag, once titles of honor for a wise old woman, have become in common language vehicles for derision."[3] As women today step into the aging limelight, there comes the realization that we are now moving into a time in our lives that society terms as "old." People begin to treat us differently. Someone may address us in a patronizing tone as we stand in a supermarket line or arrive at a social function.

My first early experience in this regard was actually several years ago when I drove through a fast food chain restaurant at eleven o'clock at night. I had just completed a demanding six-month project at my office. Filled with satisfaction and yet nearly exhausted, I thought a cup of coffee at that late hour would be a welcome companion on my drive home. When I asked the young teenage employee how much the coffee cost, he asked, "How old are you, anyway?" It was like I was being "carded" for coffee. It seemed like an unlikely question. Initially confused, I could not imagine why he would ask. After I asked for clarification about what he meant, I began to realize in the short exchange that followed that his question was relative to qualifying me for the available senior discount. I was stunned. When I pulled away, I looked in the rearview mirror. I decided that as I was hotfooting it to fifty-five years of age at that time, I indeed looked different than the thirty-nine-year-old me that was tucked away in my memory. Granted, it was late in the day and I was exhausted. Certainly, I wasn't looking my best. However, I thought I was experiencing a case of mistaken identity. Although I want to think that the young man didn't mean any disregard, it was an experience that made me realize I was physically viewed as an older woman.

Everywhere we look, we get messages that our value as women is based on retaining youthful attributes, whatever our age and at whatever cost. This makes the aging process very difficult. Instead of freely moving with integrity into the next stage of our lives, women can become caught up in a futile struggle of denying or ignoring the reality of their own aging. Because looking like an older woman has negative consequences in the job market, socially, and in essentially every area of life, many women try to combat this natural process. Unfortunately, a preoccupation with retaining youthfulness drains energy away from a woman's inner life. It diminishes her attention to fulfilling dreams and meaningful quests, and making valuable contributions.

To change negative views of aging, we need an understanding of the realities and possibilities in the second half of women's lives. Since this is a fairly new endeavor in our culture, there are many key issues to consider. We can draw upon the wisdom of our experiences, enliven our sense of imagination, and continue to manifest new, as well as renewed, dreams. We can intentionally focus on living compassionately as we focus on our families, communities, and world concerns. Our lives will be enriched, as will the lives of others, by increasing awareness of our oneness with the natural world. As we keep alive stories of women in our familial, cultural, and global histories, we can appreciate how aspects of aging are evolving. We *can* contribute to a positive evolution.

Re-Envisioning Aging

The twentieth century was the age of youth. It was predicted that the twenty-first century would evolve into an age of maturity.[4] If we assume the prediction to be true, women have rare opportunities to be paramount in changing cultural norms. If we choose to live within the paradigm of customary social attitudes and choose to conform to traditional views of aging, we will continue to deprive our families, communities, associations, and culture of the rich, full contributions we can provide.

When we look to prior times and in other cultures, we see that elder women, crones, wise women, and sages have been respected as integral parts of the community. Even though our culture idealizes youth and early life, the reality is there are an estimated 630 million women over the age of fifty on the planet today. The majority of older persons in our culture are women. Before the beginning of our current millennium, it was projected that there would be approximately six women for every man over the age of eighty in the more developed areas of the world.[5] Projections were that nearly half of all adult women in the United States would be at least fifty years old by the year 2010.

From online Wikipedia reports on demographics in the US, as of September 2014, there were twice as many women as men at age eighty-five and older. On immersionactive.com, statistics show that by 2015, people aged fifty and older will represent 45 percent of the United States population. By 2050, it is expected that the number of Americans aged sixty-five and older will be double from its population of 2010. Women over age sixty-five are the fastest growing population in our country today. What I take from these statistics is that women have amazing opportunities to be trailblazers in creating a new story in this century.

Our statistical numbers encompass women who are daughters, sisters, mothers, grandmothers, aunts, wives, partners, professionals, and businesswomen. We are caregivers, pet owners, community volunteers, neighbors, and various community and world leaders. We are women who have had many roles, obligations, and skill sets, and still do. We are significant to our families, and valuable to our communities and the world. Isn't it truly time to question our society's view of us as older women? Is it relevant to reframe what has been the socially determined and dispensable time of life?

As we step actively into this important social issue and examine what has previously been the socially accepted aging process, it becomes even clearer that aging has been, and still is, viewed as a less-than-desirable experience. Our society begins early with cynical cards, jokes, gestures, and insinuations toward those who attempt to celebrate birthdays from their mid-years on. I recall my sister-in-law, Patty, receiving a dozen dried black roses on her fortieth birthday, supposedly an elegant joke. Men are certainly not exempt. My friend, Ken, received a cane with a horn attached to it for his fiftieth birthday. One might think these acts are all in fun. However, when we look at the underbelly of what has typically been accepted, *successful aging* has been considered as nothing more than gracefully slowing the inevitable decline of the body and the mind.

Aging is generally considered an unfolding of diminishing returns. Expectations have been clear. Life has been considered a big "bell curve" at best—one long incline to a plateau of physical virility, potent sexuality, fertility, and productivity. Then, if we are lucky, we begin a slow decline after menopause, continuing throughout the second half of life, and on to our finish line. Do you see this as an inviting concept?

As I have worked closely with older individuals for many years, I have witnessed their lives differently. Sociologist William Sadler's observations are consistent with what I have seen, and what I have also personally experienced. He believes the reality is that life is a series of "sigmoid curves" that involves perpetually rising to a peak in our lives which is then followed by yet another decline.[6] Life is an ongoing series of endings and beginnings with unavoidable chaos in the transitions between *not anymore* and *not quite yet.* We have endless possibilities before us for amazing new chapters yet to unfold, and as many as we can possibly conjure until our last breath. As far as I see, it is up to each of us to grab on to this reality as our vision!

It is truly unfortunate that so many desperate efforts and exorbitant amounts of money continue to be expended in attempts to turn back the time of life. I wonder if those of us over the age of fifty really want to return to our past. At what point do we take off the mask of denial and accept that the beauty of aging is not defined by youthful physical aspects? As women, taking off that mask is difficult in a culture that begins to see us as transparent when our hair turns white, when our facial creases become more prominent, and when we become rounder in our bellies.

I interact with older women every day and am astonished when I consider all of the fascinating and diverse life experiences we inclusively have to offer. I believe that maturing women have fire in their hearts to live with deeper intention and passion. Many are amazing examples of living with authentic purpose; others are hoping yet to discover their voice and actions of unique expression. Whether we are in the second half of life, in what is called the third phase, or even the last stage of life, we can choose to add life to our days, and life to the planet. So let's take the frontlines and challenge stereotypical norms!

When historical messages of aging are confronted, the context can begin to change as we implement tools of discovery. Essential to the process of creating a shift in our viewpoints is to recognize and claim the great depths of wisdom we have gained from decades of living and learning. This recognition alone begins to cement a foundation to build a new exemplar—a new life-giving model. Women coming together to bring voice to their personal issues and experiences encountered throughout their sixth, seventh, eighth, ninth, and even tenth decades can provide powerful grounding as we begin to unearth a new cultural context. Wouldn't that be an amazing beginning point?

The grand news is that the second half of life does offer some of the richest and most rewarding decades we, as women, will experience. What once was considered the peak of our lives in the midyears is clearly shifting due to our increasingly extended lifespan and courageous choices to make the best of the voyage. What was viewed as a time of lessening contributions is now becoming viewed as an era of vibrant opportunities. As we integrate liberating images of aging, encourage change, and explore new models of development, we can more fully contribute to our communities at a time when global issues require all the wisdom humanity can impart.

Birthing a New Story

The annual Sage-ing® International Conference was recently held in Seattle. The focus of the conference was Gifting the World as We Age. As I shared with my audience the seminar topic of "Birthing Wisdom in the Second Half of Life," I was enthralled to be part of a movement that was intent on birthing a new story. It was clear that the conference was a cauldron for simmering novel ideas, creative notions, out-of-the-box insights, and potent hope for the world at large. People who gathered there were in the second half of life.

I spoke personally with many who understood that more meaningful experiences are possible as we recognize that fulfillment can be manifested when we live from the center of our wise spirits. Of course, the natural unfolding of building new visions and extending our gifts and contributions is indeed creating cultural transformation. As transformation evolves, both women and men gain greater awareness of their significant potential to gift the world, personally, locally, and globally in extraordinary ways.

Seniors at the Sage-ing® International Conference realized that we have reached a critical time in our culture in which we are called to reassess outmoded paradigms. The typical context of aging must be reassessed from a mature and soulful perspective. We are at the crossroads of an evolutionary new story relative to what maturity involves. Certainly, it is exciting to consider that women are central to the creation of a new mythos as we "re-weave" the tapestry of our own lives. Our individual context shapes our vision of life, including aging and the choices we make throughout our life duration. What we discover and model will absolutely affect future generations.

As we intentionally unearth new ways of living fully in our later years, progress of evolving into a higher level of consciousness will not be deterred. However, if we continue to hold onto rules that have previously governed us, evolution will be stalled. We co-create change and growth by releasing prior conventions when appropriate. As we begin to focus on possibilities, we must acknowledge that the script for such transformation is incomplete, emerging, and perpetually fluid. Emergence of cultural transformation not only requires embracing a new vision, but also requires courage to live through significant transitions in our personal lives that are inherent to change.

Potentially, a different kind of personal growth is vital to transform our societal views. We can initiate a new and rich vision of living our lives fully by acknowledging our physical, mental, emotional, and spiritual capacities. I also believe that a new consciousness of aging means gathering and manifesting the enormous positive potential that each of us has for growth, love, happiness, and generativity. Expanding our potential also involves living with purpose and passion.

It is prudent to understand that a new vision cannot be fully developed instantaneously—it takes time. However, we can begin by renewing our sense of imagination, drawing upon the rich wisdom of our own unique experiences, and taking in the stories of other women. As we embrace liberating self-images and identify individual and unique ways of maturing, we create impetus to transform legacies in our families and for generations yet to be birthed.

Our experiences as aging women of today are distinctly different than the experiences of aging women in prior generations. Furthermore, our probable extended life spans will generate opportunities not previously possible to create intergenerational healing and evolution. Our "culture's story" of aging—the expectations and stereotypical images of aging—does not have to be our story. Women's aging can be embraced and celebrated as our sacred journey of emerging wisdom!

Awakening the Wise Spirit

As women begin to tackle what has previously been the socially accepted aging paradigm and pursue a new model of maturity, we will also need to create liberating images, practices, and lifestyles. Isn't it true that the most meaningful change begins within our own personal lives? Therefore, in reframing our own aging, we start by studying with loving eyes the views we have of ourselves, the way we live our lives, and the manner in which we view the world. As we gain new insights, we can then positively transform views and practices by recognizing and claiming the wisdom we have gained throughout our decades.

A few years ago, I attended a class at Wisdom University in San Francisco. Students examined the relationship between wisdom and civilization, culturally and personally, relative to the book, *The Cultural Creatives*.[7] Generally described, "Cultural Creatives" are individuals in our culture who have interest in living with personal authenticity. Authors Paul Ray and Sherry Anderson emphasized the importance of women as they lead the way in this new subculture. To clarify further, the underlying themes of this subculture, a "Wisdom Culture," include serious ecological and planetary interests, emphasis on relationships and women's perspectives, and commitment to spirituality and psychological development. They have disaffection with the large institutions of the modern era, including right and left politics, materialism, and status display. Cultural Creatives are integral to an emerging culture that focuses on creating a new way of living for the good of our current and future generations.

It was then that it dawned on me that my commitment to explore typical views of aging also involved examining conventional role perspectives, such as the role of "matriarch." I realized that the function of conventional roles certainly could be underscored when beneficial. It may also be valuable to expand old patterns, or release them when appropriate, and create new definitions. All is necessary for our social, emotional, psychological, and spiritual evolution, individually and as a culture. My intention was not to "throw the baby out with the bathwater," so to speak. However, it seemed imperative to look into aspects that may not be helpful for the evolution of a maturing culture.

My awareness relative to the role of matriarch would not have been so poignant before my own mother's death. Three months prior, in the early hours on that August 9th morning, I sat through the night with her in prayer. When I received similar phone calls in prior months that her health had taken yet another diminishing turn, I would immediately catapult into fast forward, organizing my life, throwing clothes in a suitcase. I would rush to board the next flight possible out of Seattle to Nebraska to be with her and my father. There was an inner knowing that particular night that my mother's time with us truly was coming to a close. An anxious peace, if there is such a thing, came over me as I contemplatively waited with her through the night, yet 1,550 miles apart. That was the night that my life, as her daughter, as a mother, an aunt, and as a woman, changed dramatically in my mind.

Immediately after my mother's death, I poignantly realized that I was the family matriarch, whatever that meant. In my mid-fifties, I was the oldest woman in my family. I hadn't even thought of that before then. During the ensuing months, I was compelled to define what that meant since the definition was seemingly so nebulous as far as I knew. Certainly, I perceived the role of the oldest living woman of a tribe to be a heartfelt and potentially serious responsibility.

Examples of matriarchs, including my mother, left me somewhat devoid of clarity of how to live from a position of family leadership that was genuine to my nature, beliefs, and values as a woman. Historically, I had seen matriarchs in my family emerge sitting quietly in the family circle like wise, silent owls surveying the family activities. There was feminine power that emerged from silence, although we could also speculate that their silence may have reflected degrees of oppression. In *Women's Ways of Knowing*, the authors describe this type of silence as "a position in which women experience themselves as mindless and voiceless and subject to the whims of external authority."[8]

Women in my family abided by unwritten "no" rules: like no cussing, no smoking, no dancing, and no infidelity. There were also the "yes" rules: worship on Sunday; provide all the duties that make the family function smoothly relative to loving care, food, and shelter; of course, participate in the larger community. I witnessed those in my family who lived deeply in the clutches of denial in order to uphold a respectable outward appearance for self and the family unit, possibly for the sake of pride, or due to guilt, or maybe influenced by religious or community opinions. Most troubling was that female leadership also came from a history of patriarchal expectations.

Loving and enduring devotion prevailed, both self-denying and self-sacrificing, for a perceived good of the family. Generally speaking, my matriarchs were "helpmates" for their spouses. Although devotion was no doubt considered a virtue, many times devotion for the needs of others was offered at the personal expense of disregarding one's own needs, desires, dreams, and aspirations. Nonetheless, such was not without honor and respect from members of the family.

From my viewpoint, my female ancestors certainly paid high prices while living according to their defined roles. When they were not consciously aware of choices they had that may have been more truly aligned with their own authentic beliefs, opinions, and desires, they automatically acted in familiar and rote ways. I am not implying that women did not make their own choices. What I am suggesting is that by living under the umbrella of unchallenged tribal expectations and not opening to authentic self-evolution, leadership potential, and hopeful possibilities, they were unfortunately thwarted. No doubt, family members have experienced great loss in this regard, although most have not even been aware of such loss. I came to realize that when elder women are devoid, on any level, of the unique magnificence of living in self-honesty as women in their own right and as authorities of their own life choices, then members of their own tribes and participants in local and global communities do not benefit from incredible depths of rich, forthright, female leadership.

Gaining greater awareness of my desire to review my own life from a wisdom perspective, I began to grapple, step-by-step, with my personal definition of matriarch. In our Western culture, there are no specific qualifications, ceremonies, or guidelines for such a role. The current definition on merriamwebster.com of *matriarch* is "a mother who is head or ruler of her family," which I dare say does not instill much clarity, guidance, or even aspiration in our culture. Furthermore, it defines a small population of women available to activate positive leadership, if that were indeed a woman's goal.

A deeper desire to discern these matters emerged following my father's sudden death fourteen months after my mother's passing. In Jane Brooks' book, *Midlife Orphan*, she explains that the life passage following the death of a second parent is when we are "no longer anyone's child."[9] However, I believe we are always the begotten legacy of our parents, and our children will likewise carry our living legacy in their bones when we are no longer living in human form. My musings about the legacy of matriarch expanded to consider the need for redefining feminine leadership, at a time when I experienced an absence of mine.

The position of a family's matriarch includes agreeing with the rules, beliefs, values, and patterns that emerge from a patriarchal paradigm. Therefore, a matriarchal role implies there is also a patriarchal role. Of course, if one no longer ascribes to a patriarchal paradigm, then a matriarchal paradigm cannot metaphorically prevail either. Neither was consistent with my own authentic views relative to a Wisdom Culture paradigm.

When I realized I could not adhere to historical models of matriarch in my family, my view of matriarch began to crumble. A new question began to emerge. I wondered whether matriarch is a concept that is a role or function. Possibly, an even greater query may be to ask how we, who are the eldest women of our families, will fulfill wise leadership functions. Eckhart Tolle encourages us to identify with a "function" without it becoming a "role." Although he was not speaking specifically to women, there is something to learn from this. Tolle states, "When your sense of self is entirely or largely derived from it, the function easily becomes overemphasized, exaggerated, and takes you over."[10]

If we let go of notions of matriarchal roles and pre-established definitions that emerged from seemingly restrictive unconscious patterns and presumptions, clearly a new definition for authentic female leadership is warranted. While matriarch implies attending to responsibilities that an eldest woman has in a family system, my concern involves identifying less confining qualifications. In other words, how do masses of women, regardless of whether they are "eligible" as matriarchs or not, consciously activate positive change on behalf of maturing women? While some women find great value in the matriarch paradigm, my hope is to expand it to a more inclusive vision. The model of matriarch may remain, become refined, or may fall on its own. Whether matriarchal or patriarchal roles are right or wrong is not the prevalent query. What may be most pertinent is our courage to step into the challenge of creating change with a new, unfamiliar, and dynamic paradigm.

The "elder," particularly in Native American culture, provides a wonderful example of revered aging. As I have interacted with the Northwest S'Klallam and Suquamish tribes for many years, it is clear that their communities recognize elders as their most valued and wise resource. What if we began to claim our position as valued resources in Western culture? We would experience greater empowerment as we opened our hearts to embrace our aging as a revered journey. In opening our hearts, I believe our critical task is to then acknowledge and claim our own authentic wisdom. I suggest that women and men alike acknowledge and continue to develop this aspect of unique intelligence. Also, if both genders were to accept responsibility to live consciously and intentionally from the center of their wisdom and inner knowing, we would gain a broader field to initiate change. Nonetheless, our efforts and contributions have potential to become significant. Change will be imminent culturally, as it is within me, as our own awareness becomes a natural change agent.

Again, the deeper enquiry is, "How can re-envisioning women's aging in the second half of life provide opportunities to enrich living by furthering their psychological, relational, social, and spiritual development?" By exploring a reframing of our own aging as women, we gain a new foundation to positively transform views and practices that have been confining. As we initiate meaningful change beginning with our own personal lives, it is important to consider views we have of ourselves, the ways we live our lives, possibilities we envision, and the manners in which we view the world. Reframing our aging will no doubt include creating liberating images, practices, and lifestyles. It also makes sense to presume that we are now called to provide leadership within our family systems and communities beginning with understanding our own unique guiding "wisdom story."

Emergence of the Sage

To create change, it is prudent to explore realities and possibilities in which women's aging can be embraced and celebrated. I believe one possibility is for women to view themselves as *sage leaders*. My definition of a "sage leader" is "any person over the age of fifty who intentionally imparts a wise mentoring spirit, is a living example of personal authenticity, and makes a conscious commitment to a compassionate, vital life-affirming second half of life." As I massaged this definition, the word *Sagessence* emerged in my thinking. I imagined this word as a derivative from *sage* meaning "wise," and *essence* meaning "spirit." Imagine that the word "Sagessence" is descriptive of the "beauty of feminine fullness illuminating from a woman living as a sage leader from her center of wisdom gained from living the sacred journey of her life." I invite you to imagine further that this woman is you. You need not be qualified by age or family status. You are qualified by your willingness, no matter what your life experiences have been.

My intention in looking through a new lens of "sage leadership" is not confined to defining and initiating "sages" specifically, although I personally believe that is essential. The initial task is to re-envision our context of aging to include an image of "woman sage." As the mass of baby boomers continues forward in their third phase of adulthood, it is clearly a critical and fertile time for a transformational shift to transpire effectively in our culture. As you personally create ongoing fulfillment in your life while embracing all aspects of aging, you can also aspire to be a woman who is called to impart untold wisdom for our time. You will not stand alone in your efforts, and you do not need to wait for an invitation.

Essentially, women sages are not acknowledged or integral in Western culture. However, dynamics of a woman sage could reflect an emerging powerful archetype. Archetypes are considered psychological structures reflected in symbols, images, and themes common to all cultures and all times.[11] Although the potential archetypal characteristics within each of us are universal, we express them differently, endowing them with somewhat different styles, traits, and mannerisms. The expression of an archetype is influenced by a person's culture, setting, and time in history. It also is a manifestation of a woman's individuality. By understanding a "sage archetype," we begin to comprehend the importance of our life stories. We also gain appreciation for the stories of other people's lives.

Clearly, our work as women sages encompasses what Paul Ray and Sherry Anderson describe relative to elders: "In every age, elders have one fundamental task to do for the culture. Their work is to carry the wisdom function: to speak for it, protect it, preserve it, and convey it forward for future generations."[12] This is a fundamental task. However, we must also facilitate change for greater emotional, social, and spiritual development for our families and beyond. Significant change begins within the heart and mind as we remain willing and open to our evolving development and maturity.

The sage helps us as we live out our own stories authentically. As humans with divinity inborn, I believe we all have the spark of "Divine wise sageness," the dynamics of which we are responsible to awaken and bring to life. As we begin to define a paradigm of living in alignment with our sageness, we also begin to identify positive and innovative contributions we can make to our families, communities, and universally while also experiencing personal fulfillment.

As emerging forms of woman sage leadership develop within our culture, we need to open our hearts to create more conscious ways of living. For example, at a celebration of Compassion in Action a few years ago in Seattle, His Holiness the Dalai Lama urged participants to rise to the challenge of creating a more compassionate world. Specifically, he urged women to step to the forefront and lead from their natural compassionate nature. He underscored that it is critical for us to do just that. We are called to unlimited opportunities and commitments, from helping children grow up happy, kind, and loving, to expanding our contributions in world leadership. As I sat in the audience holding my eighteen-month-old granddaughter in my arms that day, I took the Dalai Lama's summons seriously with heartfelt intention.

Women sages must first examine their own lives, and identify areas as well as interests that would inspire others. A question to ask ourselves may be, "How do I provide examples in my living that help others live wisely?" Or, "What more of my life can I share with others that might be of value to them?" We may wonder, "What dynamics would consciously and intentionally model wisdom to effect positive differences for our next and future generations?"

There is a powerful principle for manifesting woman sage leadership in our society. The principle is to live as if it is already so. If you desire a more harmonious global community, aspire to create harmony in your own personal life. If you desire acceptance of diversity worldwide, become

keen to your own judgments and do your personal work to
dismiss them from your own attitudes and behaviors. As
a wise woman, be open to candidly examine how you will
impart a wise mentoring spirit, how you can be a living
example of personal authenticity, and create your best life-
affirming second phase of womanhood.

Consider possibilities for yourself as a woman sage
leader. Imagine what would change if you fully embraced
your Sagessence, or wise spirit. As you consider redefining
your journey, contemplate images in the following poem
that reflect my own emerging story:

Birth of the Sage

Unlike mother's third babe,
I am now taller with breadth.
I speak my own language,
articulate and confident.
Tracings of age etch my face.
Both palms are now carved
with deep lines of a lifetime.
My heart, under fuller breasts,
nurtures dreams for the world.

Belly now supple, round—
with fullness suggesting yet
another kind of birthing,
I look into the reflection
of my mirrored naked body
uncertain of what is beyond
this incarnate illumination.
It is as if I have conceived

a life I am yet meant to live.

Inside I hear whispers
from a soft, husky voice—
Your time has come.
Let go, surrender to the
powerful pulsing rhythm
urging birth of your sage.
Reconcile the blueprint
of your life, and beget the
path of your woman soul.

Now with womanly fullness,
I sense the inner push of
a profound metamorphosis.
I summon my keen intuition,
open my well-traveled heart,
and claim seasoned wisdom
of a matured woman cloaked
in years of refined texture and
intricate tapestry of a sacred life.

Once again,
I am filled
with another
first precious breath,
and now
I know
my long-awaited sage
has been given
her birth.[13]

Whether or not you have ever given birth to a child, the underlying story of birthing can be viewed as a preparatory metaphor in readying you to allow new creations to come through your body and mind. It is fascinating that many maturing women share experiences of gaining greater depths of sensitivity, intuition, and creativity after menopause. We can claim these gifts as ongoing as we become more attuned to our life cycles, and familiar with our wisdom that has evolved and will continue to evolve throughout our phases and stages.

As we move from an age when our wombs had potential to nourish creations with life-giving water, into a post-menopausal stage, metaphorically, heat strikes fire deep in our hearts. It is from that rich place that new passions and causes are brought forth. A deeper sense of wisdom emerges from this fertile heart-centered maturity. It is through recognizing the ever-transforming nature of feminine maturation, our unique rhythms, and capacity to be inspired that we gain the capability to experience expansive significance.

Furthermore, when we view our personal evolution as a sacred journey of perpetual endings, transitions, and beginnings, we gain inspiration to live fully our expanding potential from our infrastructure of wisdom. Therefore, as you begin to grasp the depth of intelligence you have gained from years of living, and understand that rich insights will perpetually emerge, you may begin to truly recognize the wise spirit that longs to ignite in your heart. I like to think of this as a spark that waits to be activated into flame, and a potential flame that wants to be on fire. It becomes a fire in your heart that cannot be ignored. It hungers to burn.

The metamorphosis of your wise spirit asks you to

courageously open wholly to intentional psychological, emotional, mental, and spiritual development. Once you acknowledge the potency of your sagacity after it has been fallow for years, a fertile potency will begin to ignite. It is like lighting your altar candle in the dark. Imagine that.

Remember, aging can be viewed as the evolving of a woman's development into her fullness, deepening true wisdom, and entering her period of mastery. Other traditions that acknowledge the way of the wise woman provide exemplary images of older women and their evolution. When we integrate the wisdom of other traditions, we can identify ways we can also become midwives, medicine women, healers, teachers, and leaders of ceremonies. We can unleash and revel in our humor. Our focus can expand to furthering the well-being of the planet and cosmos. As our wise spirits emerge into the light of authentic woman sage leadership, we can discover new ways to walk our sacred paths with beauty, balance, and spiritual power. We can integrate this vision that is utterly compelling in its rich presentation of maturing women as sage leaders.

As a sage leader drawing from your well of wisdom, you will begin to recognize the beauty and grace that your life reflects. Regardless of your accomplishments and failures, paths taken or not, valleys or mountaintops, you can claim the name of sage. As you fully embrace the rich tapestry of your years, consciously live your life authentically, impart a wise mentoring spirit, and commit to compassionate, vital life-affirming ways of sharing life on this planet, you are called to a personal responsibility of fully revealing your Sagessence, or wise spirit.

My hope is that you are beginning to sense that you *do*

hold the key to the powerful emergence of your own wise sage. I encourage you to consider and discern your life in this new paradigm. As you move into "fertile maturity" as a sage, you will become an alchemist. The power of alchemy is the power to be a transformational author of your own life in ways that you dream and choose, positively influencing your family, community, and the world by sharing your unique endowments.

Four Fires of Sagessence

If you are seeking a new vision of aging, the timing may be perfect to embark on a new and exciting journey metaphorically embodying the "Four Fires of Sagessence." Themes within each of these elements will provide inspiring opportunities to create a distinct shift from typical paradigms of aging.

As an evolving wise woman, you may have asked, "Where will I find fulfillment and purpose in my aging?" Your answers may be found in how you express your personal authenticity, how you make vital life-affirming choices, how you live a compassionate life, and how you impart the wisdom of your years. Certainly, your discoveries will be of benefit to your children, your grandchildren, and your communities, both locally and globally. These themes hold elements to light fire in your heart that will transform your ideas, values, and choices. Believe that you will begin an inspiring transformation as you explore the vast possibilities that can theoretically arise from the Four Fires of Sagessence. Elements within these paths have potential to rouse you to new depths and perspectives. Let's look a little closer at the possibilities:

The *Fire of Authenticity* ignites our genuine truth, expands our unique creative potential, nurtures imagination to birth ideas and dreams, and inspires liberating images of our lives.

The *Fire of Passion* invites us to live passionately in the moment, to foster love, joy, wonder, and gratitude, to deepen pleasures in our living, and to make vital, life-affirming choices.

The *Fire of Compassion* stirs us to practice loving kindness, to live in the flow of loss, grief, and change, to graciously give and receive care, and to move through life transitions confidently.

The *Fire of Vision* calls us to create a living legacy that supports greater good, to manifest deeper fulfillment, to impart a wise, mentoring spirit, and to honor intergenerational connectedness.

Imagine living as a woman of wisdom embodying the Four Fires of Sagessence. Allow yourself to accept that you are a wisdom figure in a new vision of aging. It is essential to recognize the wisdom of your years, regardless of your age or life experiences. There is a wealth of understanding and knowledge that resides within you and qualifies you as a sage. By fathoming this, you will gain greater awareness of your amazing and significant storehouse of promise to create a richer and more meaningful life throughout your years.

As a sage leader, you may begin to recognize events in your life weaving in and through the Four Fires of

Sagessence. The nature of human existence does not allow us to stay in any particular aspect indefinitely. However, as we move fluidly from one life experience to another, we are likely to be immersed more so in one path than another. Yet we may—and probably will—experience ongoing transformation in our lives with the interweaving of more than one path at a time.

Therefore, as you begin to imagine a vast potential that is waiting to be ignited in your life, hold a vision of having faith in yourself and your inner knowing. Remember your unique spark of life. Trust your truth and your insights. Have courage to continue creating your best life, for yourself, for those you love, and for the world. Seek to understand the depths of your unique gifts as you live fully the magnificence of your Sagessence. As you embody these symbolic fires, and acknowledge and celebrate the emergence of your inner sage, you will manifest richer and more significant experiences throughout your second phase of womanhood.

It is helpful to hold an image of "waking up" as fundamental to developing radical changes in our lives, and the culture at large. Similar to spirituality, it can be viewed as developing an art of wakefulness, which involves the art of being awake, of being aware, conscious, and alive.[14] Indeed, this is what we can aspire to as we review our sacred journeys, embrace changing views of aging, and live fully from the center of our wisdom. It is the art of living the truth of our lives and inner knowing.

Integrating the theme of waking up, we begin to understand that all aspects of living in later decades are permeated with Divine presence and continue to be perpetually pregnant with Divine potential. Our sacred life journey encompasses the art of living this truth and includes all our concerns, relationships, and challenges. Therefore, regardless of experiences, opportunities, or obstacles faced, we can live more fully by consciously and perpetually waking up and rising to our Divine potential. We then can begin to create new dynamic images to effect meaningful reform.

Personal fulfillment can deepen as we awaken and become more intentional in embracing the Four Fires of Sagessence and visualizing a sacred path of aging. It is life-giving to awaken to the Divine presence everywhere and especially in our aging. Our potential for compassionate, vital, life-affirming choices during this time of life rises to the surface of our consciousness as we open to new visions. A radical change in cultural views requires an awakening in our hearts and minds relative to our ways of living as we engage in reformative action.

I encourage women, who yearn for change, to awaken to the process of discerning their vision as a sage. We can be certain that everything is at stake at this time, in this century. To create cultural transformation, new visions and contributions in the second half of life, individually and in community, will greatly affect our future. Our own well-being is clearly essential to the health of society.

We are called to keep faith in our new visions. As we keep faith in new dreams, we have the opportunity to live the most meaningful lives ever lived on Earth. And as conscious sage leaders, we will continue to gain greater insight into opportunities for abundant personal fulfillment. Thereby, we will be influential in generating momentous conditions for the greater good in this generation and future generations.

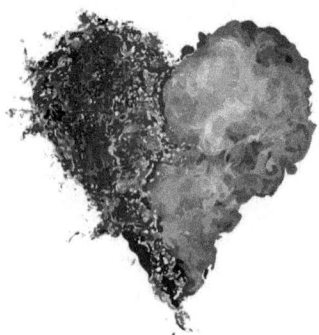

Chapter 2

The Fire of Authenticity

♥

Fire of Authenticity
**ignites our genuine truth,
expands our unique creative potential,
nurtures imagination to birth ideas and dreams,
and inspires liberating images of our lives.**

The foundation of the Four Fires of Sagessence is grounded in the heart of a woman's personal authenticity, and is core to the *Fire of Authenticity*. The Fire of Authenticity is essential, and it ignites our truth. Authenticity means truthfulness. If we are authentic, we cannot be false. Therefore, authenticity means to remain true to our being. It calls for us to always listen to our inner voice and to follow its guidance, no matter what our age. It is essential that we always respect our emotions and feelings. Remember, when we are congruent inside and out, our faces and actions will tell our truth.

Authenticity beckons us to expand boundaries of what is possible as our decades unfold. It invites new and liberating visions in our imaginations. Through self-trust and resourcefulness, we discover inspiring ways to bring our ideas and dreams to reality. It is from our position of authenticity and personal truth that our unique creative potential and boundless ingenuity gives depth to the tapestry of our life.

To live fully, we must be open to continuing our journey into all that we can be. This calls us to become intimate with our own emerging desires with self-honesty and to turn away from any age-old self-defying actions. This may require us to look at our lives for "truths" that no longer resonate with our understanding and discernment, and to be willing to move into unexplored territory.

Throughout the ebb and flow of life, women sages are able to uphold their genuineness and live courageously moment by moment. Sages have the capacity to hold the tension of the creative process, which is actually active in the unfolding of each moment. They trust their imagination and ideas to bring solutions to light. These are women who become masters of manifesting their own fulfillment while also honoring an interconnectedness with all living things.

Igniting Genuine Truth

Although status for mature women in our society does not exist, women do describe that there are points as they become older when they feel as though they have come into their own. Many women spend years preserving relationships and lifestyles and being dedicated to maintaining them. Then, in their maturing years, women tend to become more assertive and willing to encounter challenges or risk loss in order to follow their own truth and priorities. They learn to live more authentically and balance the needs of self with those of others. Many elderly women become more capable, authoritative, and diverse at a time of life when experiences of change become more prevalent.

As we experience change in elder years, endings often create a return to new beginnings. As women, we can birth newness again and again even in our aging. We can perpetually experience a self-awakening and birthing of self. I believe new beginnings provide the impetus to experience this awakening: a rebirth of oneself and one's subsequent fruitfulness. With the realization of our oneness with an omnipresent sacredness—regardless of how we name that presence, we can begin to grasp that we are involved in a perpetual and ongoing co-creative process.

New beginnings provide opportunities to discover hope, grace, and blessing. Essentially, new opportunities can potentially become catalysts to capture deeper layers of personal authenticity and identify lost aspects of ourselves, perhaps buried for years. We may recognize a gap between an inner sense of potential (that is who we once were and/or wanted to be) and who we have become. Perhaps we remember earlier strengths and aspirations that were lost in our adult life. By reclaiming previous aspects or by acknowledging newly discovered passions, we create incentives for nurturing our dreams and living more fully into our authentic sense of self.

I recall a lively, intelligent woman who was a patient of mine. When I first met Ruth, I was amazed by her astonishing presence. She dressed in long, flowing layers of colorful material and textures, wore large multicolored eyeglasses, and her lips were glazed with bright orange lipstick to match her long curly, flaming red hair. She spoke in a confident, articulate, bold manner. I learned this lovely woman had not always been so gregarious. She had lived in the shadow of her husband's profession as a minister for years. After he passed away, she began college classes and in her late sixties completed a PhD. At the time I met Ruth, she was teaching courses in human sexuality at a local university and at off-campus military sites. Ruth shared with me, "I scare my students sometimes with my candor. They are surprised that I am not shocked by any question, and seem to be amazed that I have helpful insights. They appreciate talking with me about sexuality." With a mischievous glimmer in her eyes, she added, "I really can give them something to think about!" It was amazing to see this woman, then in her late seventies, so full of life-giving energy. She was a woman who had recognized her potential, nurtured her dreams, and redefined her elder years of living. Ruth was a fine example of personal authenticity.

One of our greatest challenges is to live authentically from the wise spirit that resides within, to create our lives anew, and celebrate unceasingly. As women sages, we live more fully into our own authenticity by celebrating our strengths and understanding our weaknesses. We rely on our fortes over and over again, recognizing them as gifts to share with others. We are genuine in creating our own lives by clarifying our desires, our passions, our hopes, and our dreams. Women sages understand there is no one else better qualified to ascertain promptings of their heart than they are personally.

Consciously living from the center of personal authenticity requires sages to shed layers of cultural, regional, and familial expectations. As we live authentically, we learn to disappoint others and speak our truth even in difficult situations. Most female children have been raised to consider other people's opinions as more significant than messages from their own heart. As sages, we must model to our children and grandchildren how we make wise choices, without guilt being a driving force, and with assurance that disappointing others typically is not as problematic as we imagine. Although disappointing others is sometimes a result of living our lives authentically, we can still choose to act with loving kindness and sometimes with tough love. Furthermore, we must cultivate the ability to make peace with disappointment and listen to our own inner voice, while honoring the voices of others. When we attune our lives to the Divine's guidance, our inner knowing is what counts.

Over recent years, I have spent my birthday week typically by myself, and by choice. Although the way I choose to create this time isn't typical to the tradition of my immediate family, they usually join me for a couple of days during my hiatus. On my sixty-first birthday, a few years ago, I spent another treasured personal "sabbath week" in one of my favorite places, the city of Victoria on Vancouver Island in Canada. This trip has become one of my savored and celebrated self-care rituals. I luxuriate in solitude and contemplation, walk the bluffs above the Strait of Juan de Fuca, browse through shops, and poke around to find new ethnic tastes. It is a time that I read and write to my heart's content. I sleep whenever my body wants. I sit on the harbor benches in the early autumn mornings, watch the fall fog lift and the sun break through. I take whatever time it takes to soothe my heart as I muse over the simplest reflections moving across the water.

One afternoon, I sauntered into one of my favorite bookstores, Munro's Books. The book, *intimacy : Trusting Oneself and the Other* by Osho immediately caught my eye.[1] Before I left the store, I had purchased the book as a birthday gift for myself. I bought a cup of coffee and began to read. I was enthralled with the philosophy of this spiritual teacher. His words kept running through my mind. Essentially, he encourages us to trust ourselves and come to "know the beauty" of trusting—the serenity, calmness and quietness that emerges. Osho believed that the more we trust ourselves, others, and even the *unknown*, the more we activate deep serenity, calm and quiet in our *beingness*. Most beautiful in this way of life is that the more you and I practice trust, the grander we *soar* in our lives—positively affecting our very core and others around us, and affecting constructive change in ways in which we may never become even remotely aware.

I thought, certainly this is central to the message of the Four Fires of Sagessence, and specifically the Fire of Authenticity. We must trust ourselves and pursue a deeper understanding of what self-intimacy is all about as we consciously live the elements of this path and let its fire come to life.

Expanding Creative Potential

Many women find that the second half of life becomes their most richly creative and inspiring decades. How marvelous to continuously discover and create regardless of our life circumstances. When we become aware of passions or dreams that reside within our heart, we can then begin to name them. In naming what we dream, we rouse whatever it is and then it is our responsibility to nurture what it wants to become. Freeing our creative potential with refreshing ideas and notions, no matter what, bestows us with gifts of fulfillment.

Innovative vitality that emerges during the second half of life is a process of coming to personal fullness. From this perspective, aging is a ripening, a coming to fruition. In coming into our fullness, there is a necessity to be open to the creative tension that emerges from knowing how our life has evolved to the present and what we now want to become. Discernment becomes essential and requires close listening to the inner creative urges and imaginings. Liberating our ingenious potential is powerful.

Hildegard von Bingen, a fifteenth century mystic, taught that all creation and humanity is "showered with greening refreshment, and vitality to bear fruit."[2] Her concept of *viriditas* or *greening power* relates to our creative power. As a woman's greening power emerges, she learns to trust her intuition. She fosters her imaginations and brings creativity into form.

Unfortunately, many women internalize societal messages of aging and use age as a factor in limiting their creative choices. Age is an imperfect measure of human energy and capability. We need not live out the span of our lives like the bell curve. We are not moving away from a potent era of creative potential mid-span. We need not experience the last phase of womanhood as an era of increasing diminishment to our end. In reality, our rhythm of life flows time and again into new, rich opportunities of diversity, particularly in our creativity.

Creating our best life calls us to continue personal development and take time to discover our creative gifts. We may choose to separate from our old lifestyles and values. We may also separate from personal belongings, relationships, and/or professions that do not support our authentic interests or the ongoing healthy existence of the inhabitants of the world and its environments.

Indeed, our creative potential is a vast field before us. As we explore new creative expressions, we can open ourselves to experience inspiration through gardening, mentoring, meditation, dreamwork, writing, teaching, body prayer, spiritual pilgrimages, and volunteering. Through the creation of poems, legends, mosaics, carvings, handwork, paintings, songs, dance, music, and sculptures, sages make the world stand still long enough for others to glimpse its mystery. We can learn to play a musical instrument, write poetry, return to school for a degree, fall in love again, make new friends, or change careers. Works of art are the fruit of the imagination. The imagination keeps alive a mysterious and sacramental vision of life. Age itself does not set these limits. Women in their sixth, seventh, and eighth decades are doing all of these.

Arts that have been lost—such as rituals, ceremony, play, storytelling, and a deep sense of collaborative community— can be reclaimed, valued, and supported by women sage leaders. We can integrate various expressions of art into our lives. This is not only for cultural inspiration but also as a means to nurture sensory development, personal growth, and expression, as well as spiritual practice. At a time when women seek outlets for their creative energy that are more satisfying, they also integrate their creativity with their deep concern for the state of the world. They desire to live their lives fully and discover ways to further share their talents. Many women discover vocations that advance the well-being of the planet.

Play and humor are also aspects of the imagination and

vital to our aging. As some of our responsibilities recede, we have time to enter again into those attitudes that liberate creative powers such as wonder toward life, a sense of discovery, the capacity for leisure, and freedom to play. These provide opportunities to notice things more vividly and deeply.

I am reminded of a woman I knew as "Hedda" (not her real name), a woman in her late seventies who I became acquainted with several years ago. Before I knew Hedda's story, I was always amused by her enjoyable presence. She wore childlike clothes of stripes, dots, and primary colors. Her shoes were always a topic of discussion—usually bright red Mary Janes with a dancing heel. Once, when Hedda was in her sixties she looked in the mirror hung in her sewing room. As she gazed at the face that looked back at her, she was compelled to open a notion drawer and reach for a red pom-pom. She whimsically placed the pom-pom on her nose. Then, she studied the details of her aging face. Looking into the blue eyes that stared back at her in the mirror, she realized *that* face had been her front to the world through tears and laughter, joy and disaster. Many times in her life, sadness took over her face—sometimes for hours, days, and, sometimes it was years. She could not remember exactly at the time.

Hedda hesitantly touched her mouth reflected in the mirror. She began to smile broadly—then whimsically. Her smile was like a good friend well remembered. Sometimes her mouth smiled even when her blue eyes were sad. But in those moments, the memory of her laughing mouth reminded her that life could be full of joy. In that *aha* moment, she began to cry.

There never seemed to be a reason why Hedda's moods

changed from joy to sadness so quickly. She could go from an outburst of laughter, singing, and dancing, and then suddenly be interrupted by tears. However, that evening while looking in the mirror, she recognized "it." It was a clown! Delightfully, she said to herself, "It's time for YoYo to come out!" She danced around the small sewing room with the red pom-pom held to her nose.

Hedda put her arms around the persona of "YoYo" and integrated the role of a clown in her life. During the years that followed, Hedda clowned as YoYo at community fairs and festivals, children's clubs, and hospitals. She said she humored "old people" at senior centers, retirement homes, and care facilities. Never did she seem deterred by her own aging. It appeared that her heart became younger and younger.

Hedda traveled to Asia several times to share her passion of clowning with children in orphanages. When she became aware that her memory was failing, she decided to discontinue international travel. She began volunteering seven days a week at an Alzheimer's care facility in her local community. With more time available, Hedda also decided to learn to paint with watercolor and oils, and did so fervently and confidently. She began to write poetry. Her creative potential exploded!

Fears never daunted Hedda. After all, she had hidden in earthen holes under her parents' home during World War II. Then came imprisonment, torture, and rape in Auschwitz. When she was freed from the torment of prison, her mother insisted she flee her homeland. As a child, Hedda dreamed she would be an actress, yet she could not imagine the life she had dreamt after her teeth were all pulled as an act of torture while she was imprisoned. Her *way to freedom* was to marry an American soldier and move to the United States, leaving her mother and father in Germany. Afterward, she lost a child. Her parents died. Later, her husband was forever missing-in-action in the Korean War. There were two incidents in Hedda's life whereby she completely lost all her possessions. One time was in Germany, and the other was when fire engulfed her home in America. What had she to fear? She freely gave her gift of love and talents, shared her joy, and delighted little children. She made people laugh. Hedda embodied ingenious inspiration.

A woman like Hedda is an admirable example of a woman freeing her creative potential, no matter her age or life circumstances. It is refreshing and life-giving to understand that after years of attempting to align with other people's needs and expectations, facing various dilemmas, and moving through trials and deterrents, that a later phase of life is indeed an era when a woman's creative potential can emerge into fascinating and influential self-expressions. The possibilities are unlimited. Contributions can be far-reaching into the lives of others in ways not ever fully realized when we dare trust the creative power of our imagination.

Trusting Imagination

In the second phase of womanhood, we begin to take seriously new images that emerge in our imagination. It is vital to trust that which gestates in your soul and evolves in your imagination. As you deepen your trust in this process, you will also gain respect for the importance of fresh images that emerge into consciousness.

When a woman recognizes the wisdom of her imagination, she begins to realize the value of attending to her inner life. It is from the inner life that ideas come forth. The sage begins to understand the worth of fostering her creative process. This process always requires time for our ideas to develop and evolve. Consider the seed of a plant that evolves in fertile ground, and then emerges into the perfection of its true nature in perfect timing. Hereby, innovation is born again and again.

Deeper exploration of your inner life may result from new practices to attain awareness, discovering new or rediscovering old dreams, and connecting with inventive ideas. You can expand possibilities for your imagination to develop creatively through means of solitude, meditation, writing, and dreamwork.

Solitude. Solitude is a space or time apart, but one held and sustained by a sense of connection and peace with oneself and others. Solitude is a lovely place to bask in a quiet and nurturing space to settle your heart and mind. Leaving the frenzy and demands of outer activities and responsibilities, even for short periods of time, helps you gain room to discover your own inner depths. You can come to cherish the silence that allows clearing of mind and body in order to identify images and dreams to rise from the storehouse of your imagination.

Meditation. Meditation is a practice of clearing and calming the mind. It requires recognition of energy, both external and internal. All living matter is made of energy; meditation allows us to acknowledge energy and use it for our physical, mental, emotional, and spiritual benefits. Reading and reflecting meditatively are also vital to spiritual living and can allow us to connect to inner messages of wisdom. In the midst of all the competing values of contemporary culture, meditation nourishes, centers, and gives us direction. There are many traditions and teachings on how to practice various ways of meditation. Consider including poetry, music, walking, mandalas, finger labyrinths, painting, and photography as ways to discover deeper joy and satisfaction in this practice.

Writing. Journaling is a path to personal discovery and self-revelation. Of course, your journal actually provides a record of your life journey. It reveals the patterns, alerts you to the turning points, and reveals landscapes of your life. It also allows your ideas to be described by words. Journaling is an enduring means of finding intimacy with self and with others.

Many women find great gratification in capturing moments and experiences through poetic expression— another way of exploring inner life through an art of writing. I personally honor poetry as prayer and a spiritual practice that provides openings for healing, discernment, enlightenment, and celebration. Poetry is a way of giving the soul voice. Whether a poet is seasoned in the art or not, inimitable words and unique meanings reflected in all poetry can only be delivered through each writer's authentic life and by her soul's voice. Therefore, poetry written by any woman is extraordinary and unequaled in creation.

Dreamwork. Dreams are sources of information, insight, and wholeness. Many cultures regard dreams as higher states of consciousness and as fonts of knowledge more important than those available during ordinary wakefulness. Although we typically think dreamwork is relative to night dreams, rich wisdom does emerge in a woman's daydreams as well. Explore guidance for life's passages in your dreams by attending to images that you perceive. Be sure to consider those images as sources of notable elements of wisdom to add to your plethora of imaginative assets. Remember that in this time of life, cathartic images are birthed to promote liberation.

Inspiring Liberating Images

The Fire of Authenticity calls women in the second half of life to attend to liberating images of aging. Becoming women of wisdom means opening to emerging insights; it means applying those insights to create liberating images of older women. Identifying liberating images is also essential for younger women who may be searching for mentors. To stimulate thoughts, let's explore energizing images relative to our current views of beauty, our sexuality, and spirituality. These three areas generate potent conversations for women of wisdom, and are significant for us to consider on our paths of authenticity.

Beauty. Society tells us that our value as women lies in still looking young, whatever our age. This makes the aging process frustrating, especially if a woman's identity has been tied to physical beauty. The diet, cosmetic, and cosmetic surgery industries have a large economic stake in keeping the focus on youthfulness alive. Of course, we have choices. Physical changes that come with time can be gracefully accepted, sensibly and astutely encountered, or battled endlessly—sometimes even to distorting a woman's natural beauty. One thing is for certain; a preoccupation with looking young draws our attention away from our inner life and diminishes opportunities for liberation.

Polly Kline, ninety-seven years old, clearly took exception to typical cultural views of beauty. She proclaimed, "I still don't dye my hair." Ms. Kline said that she viewed herself as a role model for women in their seventies and eighties! However, her wise advice to any woman was for each of us to follow our own conscience. She shared,

> I've had several lives. I'm not the same person I was at twenty, forty, or even sixty. When you're this old, you can reconsider your whole life. You can relive your life and understand it with a pleasure and perception not available when you first experienced it.[3]

The most compelling beauty emerges from the depth and texture of a person's life and spirit, and the face seems to carry it in a special way. Recently, I walked up to a customer service counter in a store to ask a question. While I was waiting in line for a few moments, an elderly woman standing next to me stepped over and said, "Excuse me. I just wanted to say I couldn't help but notice your face. I see a happy woman, and your eyes say you love to help people." She clarified, "Now, I'm not any psychic or anything like that. I just wanted to tell you what I see."

Very surprised at the encounter, I thanked her for taking a risk to share her thoughts. She smiled and said that she was seventy-eight years old and when she turned seventy-five, she decided to let her heart lead, and to say what she felt intuitively. I am still curious about this woman and the obvious personal transformation she referred to at the age of seventy-five. What I really appreciated was that she demonstrated to me her genuine sincerity. Furthermore, she did not speak to me about physical beauty, but heartfelt beauty.

A reframing of beauty stems from qualities that evoke

pleasure, satisfaction, and fulfillment. This beauty is a constant and resides deep within the self. No longer external, it cannot be taken away. Kathleen Fischer shared, "I cannot think of a single human being whom I have ever cherished whose appeal to me was based on youthful cosmetic attractiveness alone. As a matter of fact, I often turn in a crowded city to stare at a face on which experience has written a pattern of celebration."[4]

The rhythms of life beckon us to recognize that the unfolding of our own fullness and inner beauty accompanies a mysterious sense of "coming home to ourselves." The poem, "Home," from my book *Fire in the Well—Poetry for Women Awakening the Inner Sage*, speaks of an inner voice that beckons each of us as women:

> Come
> to that
> which longs
> for you
> to be fully home
> to all
> that you are.
>
> Your home
> awaits
> with open doors.
> The threshold flush;
> you
> need not
> stumble in.[5]

Sages know "the way home" to themselves, casting off what no longer benefits their authentic journey.

As we gaze at our changing faces and bodies, it is essential to develop a deeper sense of self-honor. As voices of society— that remind us of imperfections, chatter in our heads, maybe it is well to examine our ideas of imperfection. A beginning point may be to reframe our view of imperfections that accompany our aging process.

In trusting that our process of aging is interwoven with wisdom embedded in the Fire of Authenticity, a profound insight begins to emerge. As we look to nature, we gain an understanding of how beauty and *im*perfection are inseparable. Every tree reflects its beauty—yet up close, we can see a multitude of imperfections. The same is true for us as human beings. Every woman's body reflects incredible beauty. Yet every person's body is imperfect in some way. We are born with some imperfections and others we acquire. Our bodies show scars from the unique processes of a woman's life, such as lumpectomies, mastectomies, hysterectomies, and marks of giving birth—stillborn or alive. However, we can also acknowledge and celebrate what we may perceive as imperfections. Anything less is a choice to not respect the wonder and awe of our creation and the life we have experienced. By reframing views of imperfection, there comes a realization that the changes experienced in all of nature are truly consistent with the creative process of the Divine.

When we see ourselves growing older as a liberating creative process devoid of unreasonable ideals of youthful outer beauty, we can begin to trust that we are in an important and rewarding developmental stage of life. We become more ourselves: braver, more thoughtful, more inward, and thus better prepared than at any other life stage to develop psychologically and spiritually. However, there are no guidebooks that fully affirm the new strengths that are emerging in us as sages in this developmental stage. Nonetheless, I believe it is our responsibility to boldly claim our sageness, and live into our renewed visions. The truth of the matter is that as our population ages, older women are becoming self-reliant longer and longer. They are remaining healthy, engaged, creatively productive, and sexually active.

Sexuality. In previous generations, women have equated the end of fertility with the end of sexuality. However, now women may experience freedom from the fear of pregnancy, which can have the potential to rejuvenate a woman's sex life. She allows herself to become more sensuous than before. She appreciates the pleasures of her sexuality into her later years.

Women over fifty, menopausal and beyond, are beginning to discuss candidly previously unspoken topics of love, sex, dating, marriage, and remarriage. Typically, discussions have been among close friends and have not been openly elucidated in broader settings. As we openly talk about the cultural expectations of women's sexuality in the second half of life, we can also openly envision how we really want to regard our sexuality.

In her book, *Sex and the Seasoned Woman*, Gail Sheehy talks about a new universe of lusty, liberated women, some married and some not. She described a seasoned woman as *spicy*:

She has been marinated in life experience. Like a complex wine, she can be alternately sweet, tart, sparking, mellow. She is both maternal and playful. Assured, alluring, and resourceful. She is less likely to have an agenda than a young woman—no biological clock tick-tocking beside her lover's bed, no campaign to lead him to the altar, no rescue fantasies. The seasoned woman knows who she is.[6]

Indeed, this is a compelling description of a woman who lives passionately in the second half of her life. It defines a woman who, regardless of failures she has encountered, welcomes life with zest as well as sincerity. She is interested in remaining intimately connected and engaged.

One of the strongest connectors among older adults continues to be physical intimacy. According to information provided by the National Center for Biotechnology (ncbi. nlm.nih.gov), studies from 2011 found that 57 percent of Americans over the age of sixty are sexually active. However, here is an interesting and sobering finding: of this population of men and women over sixty who are still enjoying lovemaking, or at least kissing and cuddling, nearly half of them long for more sex.

The great obstacle to continuing sexual vitality in the second half of life is, of course, the death of a spouse. At agingstats. gov, it is reported that 24 percent of American women are widowed between ages sixty-five and seventy-five, 50 percent between ages seventy-five and eighty-four, and 73 percent at eighty-five years of age and older. The 2009 US Census Bureau data supports the finding that there is an escalation of widows after the age of sixty-five, with exponentially increasing percentages of women single over the age of eighty-five years.

Many women refuse to be celibate in their later years. Approximately 25 percent of both women and men age seventy-five or older agree that sexual activity is a critical part of a good relationship. About 25 percent of them continue to have sexual relations at least once a week, according to an American Association of Retired Persons (AARP) 2005 sexuality study (*Sexuality at Midlife and Beyond: 2004 Update of Attitudes and Behaviors*, AARP, 2005). However, a far greater number of women than men over seventy-five years of age admit they do not particularly enjoy sex at that age or that they would be quite happy if they never had sex again. Many of the latter women have been widowed and either have not found a new partner or have been discouraged by the preponderance of older men who are unavailable or who they do not consider sexually attractive. The AARP 2009 study findings were consistent with the prior 2004 survey. However, both frequency of sexual intercourse and overall sexual satisfaction had declined in later survey ratings.

Just because we are aging does not mean our sexuality vanishes. How do we consider creative sexuality when partner options are not as prevalent? A story told by Joan Borysenko gives insight into this creative aspect:

At eighty Julia is unmarried like 75 percent of the women in her age bracket. She is bothered by arthritis, particularly in the fingers of her left hand and in her knees, but is otherwise in good health as are two thirds of the women who live to be her age. She lives in a three-bedroom condominium on Boston's waterfront that she has shared with her friend Barbara, also a widow, for the past six years. Julia dates a man named Mike, a retired police officer who volunteers at the senior center that she directed until she was seventy-four, and still consults for several hours a week. She counts herself lucky to have a love life. She enjoys spending time with Mike, and their lovemaking is a welcome gift.[7]

Women who feel as if they are coming into their power are likely to have an increased interest in and appreciation of sex. Ruth Turner, age seventy-five, shared, "I just got married again. I answered an ad.... That's how I met Larry. I am his sexual fantasy. We have a wonderful life together, but we kept our separate apartments. We have more freedom that way, and of course, it's romantic as well."[8]

Women like Ruth appear vital and healthy. They feel like they are in the prime of their lives, and as if they are coming into their fullness. In contrast, women who buy into the myth that menopause is the end of their womanhood, the beginning of a rapid decline into aging, and loss of attractiveness, start to lose their vitality. Furthermore, negative feelings about menopause are a carryover from old beliefs that women are valuable only because of their ability to bear children. Such beliefs are still held by the majority of the world's population.

Gail Sheehy spoke of *Grandlove* that can be experienced in aging—a phase of trusted affection. This is a love that ranges in sexual experiences from affectionate closeness with a trusted companion to the "unexpected exuberance of seasoned sex."[9] This later life phase is more about enjoying our relationship(s) with absolute delight. However, there are times when our love stretches us to painful boundaries of acceptance and selflessness.

When pondering on unexpected situations that many times occur during a time of seasoned love, and that call us to extraordinary acts of love, we can learn priceless lessons from Alice Munro's short story, *The Bear Came Over the Mountain*. Munro shares the heartfelt love story of Grant and Fiona. A selfless quality of grandlove becomes apparent in their later marriage with Fiona's onset of dementia.

In the story, Fiona becomes a resident at a memory care home. Eventually, Grant discovers Fiona's fondness of a male resident, Aubrey, who had become her significant friend. Although Grant was her husband of fifty-some years, he became more of an acquaintance, if you will, and then like a passer-by in Fiona's life.

One day Grant found his beloved extremely upset, nearly emotionally debilitated and bedridden with grief. He learned that Aubrey's wife had taken Aubrey back to their home. Not only had Grant been discovering the elements of Grandlove all along, but the story painstakingly conveys his exploration into the very depths of his capacity to love.

The remainder of Munro's story was an account of how Grant successfully negotiated with Aubrey's wife to return Aubrey to the memory care home. Ultimately, Aubrey accompanied Grant back to the care facility. As Grant approached his wife, he said, "Fiona, I've brought a surprise for you. Do you remember Aubrey?" Fiona took a few moments seemingly to gather her thoughts and search her memory. Then Fiona stood to put her arms around Aubrey, and answered,

> "I'm happy to see you," she said, and pulled his earlobes. "You could have just driven away," she said. "Just driven away without a care in the world and forsook me. Forsooken me. Forsaken."
> He kept his face against her white hair, her pink scalp, her sweetly shaped skull. He said, "Not a chance."[10]

It seems any woman would delight in experiencing Grandlove with her long-time love—a spouse of fifty years. However, as in the story about Grant and Fiona, the definition of Grandlove may take us into exploration of new and boundless experiences of an astonishing capacity to love. It calls upon maturity, a seasoned heart, and an acquiescent attitude to support us in that journey.

Our attitudes relative to aging can largely affect our views of sexuality. Although, Western women are becoming increasingly liberated, it is well to acknowledge that liberation is indeed very recent. As shared in Alice Munro's story, there is new ground to explore. The reality is women are not settling for typical practices of sexual pleasure beginning with brief arousal and prompt climax. They are looking for deeper levels of pleasure, including sexual pleasure that can be expanded beyond traditional practices. For example, sexual pleasure with creative chakra energy and breath work can be enjoyed either with partners or singly.

Christa Schulte offers an invitation to expand our ideas regarding sexuality through Tantric practices. She states, "Tantra means the complete acceptance and weaving together of all our feelings, and the forging of creative bonds with other people. This includes liberation from the prison of polarities and transcendence of social and physical boundaries. It also means beginning with what we have and then expanding it in the direction of our possibilities."[11]

Through tantric practices, we can wrap our arms around honoring, celebrating, and cultivating our womanly sexual power. The dynamic creative energy that emerges through sexuality can be a pleasure and a source of vitality and well-being that endures for years into the second half of life. With Tantric practices, every woman can rejoice in the energy of her own sexuality, which can also be considered a spiritual practice that includes sex.[12]

Spirituality. Conventional paradigms of growing older

have been viewed exclusively from a biological perspective. Imagine efforts to envision aging as a sacred evolution when mature and young people, as well as ages in between, come together to create a new vision of our human journey. Can you visualize how inspiring the dialogues could be? Conversations on this topic could be potent as we continue to move away from society's definition of aging, and internalize new images that integrate spirituality.

Few studies on aging have included spiritual views. However, there is a consistently evolving interest in considering aging from a spiritual context. In her book, *Winter Grace*, Kathleen Fischer is a spiritual mentor in this regard. She encourages women to envision a "spirituality of aging."[13] When we view aging through a lens of spirituality, we can begin to see how our efforts may change as we deal creatively with retirement and attempt to find renewed purpose in our later decades. Our losses, ranging from a move from a home of many years to the death of a loved one, involve spiritual aspects. Whether we wrangle with questions of self-worth, fear of reaching out to make new friends, or declining health, our life stages are spiritual concerns. Every discovery, whether it is a new talent, deeper peace, or an expansive awareness of love, is steeped in aspects of spirituality.

Of course, spirituality is a broad concept with room for many perspectives. In general, it includes a sense of connection to something larger than we are individually. It typically involves a search for meaning in life. I have heard people describe spiritual experiences as simply a deep sense of aliveness and interconnectedness with all things. Although our views may differ about a definition, it is clear that it is a universal human experience—something that touches us all.

The second half of life is a time when many women

deepen in their spiritual practices. Some will continue to find that practices of their faith communities enrich their lives, and provide greater strength and satisfaction in their daily life. Yet there are other women who will seek other religious and/or spiritual practices. Although religious traditions may have been unquestioned throughout previous generations of a woman's history, many women at this mature time of life develop a strong sense to define their own experiences aside from scripted practices. Those may redefine spirituality in ways to connect with meaningful, nurturing spiritual experiences.

Spiritual autonomy need not separate us from our faith community, unless we choose a self-imposed hiatus from conventional religion in search of personal discernment. In that case, it is entirely likely that we may not return to our previous faith community. However, if we do rejoin a spiritual community, it is highly possible that it will need to be a supportive choice and spiritually affirming for our ongoing and evolving spiritual nurturance. What becomes imperative is that we come to trust our own personal spirituality. It is essential that we trust our own experience of the Divine, whether we are members of a faith community, are students of spiritual teachers, whether we companion with a mentor, or seek nurturing discernment singly. Nonetheless, sages increasingly intuit the high value of their individual spiritual experiences. Maturity calls forth personal responsibility to be fully present in our unique Divine happenings and spiritual journeys.

Possibly, you may come to question religious dogma and altogether consider departing from conventional practices prevalent in prior generations. This would be a time of ultimate courage, when there may be no blueprint to follow other than your own unique spiritual understanding and life path. With heartfelt doubt, you may find yourself departing from religious entrancement, stepping across an invisible threshold, and venturing from prior scripting in, many times, less-than-graceful ways. However, how it happens does not especially matter. What does matter is that you take the next step in your life journey in response to the prompting of your heart.

As we expand our consciousness, we may witness and experience the increasing presence of the Divine Feminine in our lives. In her book, *She Who Is*, Elizabeth Johnson discusses an image of One who suffers with Her beloved creation.[14] She wrote that "Spirit-Sophia" is our source of transforming energy; she initiates change and transforms what is complete into new life. Thus, in the feminine way, a transformation is manifested.

Some women seek to integrate maternal principles of the Divine Feminine. This is reflected in the poem, "Magdalena," from *Fire in the Well*:

> It took a long time . . .
> a very long time
> to finally jump off the ship
> freighted with spoon-fed theology
> and mindless doctrines.
> I told the captain of patriarchy,
> the man of vengeance and judgment,
> I had to find a god who looked like me.
> If I was going to wrangle with life,
> I wanted one of those
> busty, voluptuous wooden women
> nailed to the front of ships

to save me.
I wanted one of those
weathered, courageous females
who unflinchingly
presses into unpredictable storms
with her long, painted wood skirts
whipped back in the wild gale.
I wanted one of those
beautiful carved figureheads
to come alive,
to come to my rescue,
to hold me in her strong arms,
let me rest between her broad knees
as I shed tears in her buxom breasts,
take my hand with her sturdy grasp
and ride with me on the seas
confidently
while together we navigate
toward the harbor
of the Divine Feminine
shining bright Her beacon
across the rambunctious swells,
until we hear Her voice
shouting out, *"Come! Here I am!*
Your Magdalena!
I will give you shelter.
I will give you peace.
I will give you wisdom.
Welcome home
to a god who looks like you!"[15]

If you prefer maternal images, consider the image of "World Mother"—the glorious Divine Being that many ancient cultures, nations, and great world faiths have recognized and honored. She embodies all the highest attributes of feminine aspects in perfection, both of the creative deity and the human race. From a vantage point of world mythology, Geoffrey Hodson describes the World Mother, "She, the all-compassionate One, gazes with infinite tenderness and concern upon life on earth."[16] Another maternal image is Quan Yin, a maternal goddess who looks upon the world with compassion. She is considered One who hears all things, and encourages us to see her qualities in our own nature, so that we can also bring peace and tranquility to the world. Maternal spiritual principles may be inviting as we give ourselves over to experiencing the Divine in our own personal ways.

Sages respect the many ways women integrate spirituality into their lives. Rev. Dr. Lauren Artress, an Episcopalian priest in San Francisco, prefers to not use academic definitions of spirituality as she believes they have little practical application.[17] Women typically seek practices and teachings that help Spirit, God, Divine, or whatever name personally significant, to permeate every moment of their lives.

As we discover new spiritual meaning and purpose, let us also remember that we are spiritual examples for our children and grandchildren. We are responsible for conveying that their lives are spiritually connected in tandem with the continuous unfolding of the Universe. A child's worldview, character, and outlook for expanding possibilities are influenced significantly by their own experiences of spirituality. It is paramount for them to feel connected to all of nature, and to the extent of the cosmos. The following lyrics to *Granddaughter's Lullaby*, a song that I composed for my granddaughter before she was born, reflects cosmological teachings:

> With a burst of light
> Fragments scattered
> Gathering up stardust
> Here's my life
> . . . here's my life.
>
> And since that bright star
> Held in Sacred arms
> Transformed by your love
> Here's my life
> . . . here's my life.
>
> And I thank you
> Yes, I thank you
> I thank you for the stardust
> That's my life.
>
> And I thank you
> Yes, I thank you
> I thank you for the stardust
> That's my life.
> That's my life.
> That's my life.[18]

It is essential that we instill in each child an inner essence that propagates continuous Divine mysteries and miracles.

Lauren Artress teaches that if we are on a spiritual

path—any path from the rich traditions of the world's religions—to live a healed and transformed life, we are called to a) deepen our compassion, b) lessen our judgments, c) increase our patience, and d) find our purpose and share it with the world.[19] These four guidelines are ideals. We may never develop all of them fully, but they point in the direction we may want to go. These ideals can help us gauge our spiritual growth by reflecting on questions Artress poses:

1. Have I deepened my compassion for my family, my friends, and the strangers who cross my path?
2. Have I lessened my judgments about my loved ones and those I meet?
3. Have I increased my patience with my loved ones and those I meet?
4. Have I found my purpose, and nurtured it, so I can be of service to the world?

Another encompassing question to ask ourselves is, "Have we given life to our spiritual practice with our actions?" We can also consider what may block these ideals from becoming a deeper part of our lives.

In addition to deepening understanding of our spiritual direction, women are becoming increasingly aware that their bodies are absolutely holy. In and through our bodies we know much that is essential to human life. This is a paradox that accompanies our aging. Interior awareness often becomes richer while physical abilities slowly lessen. However, we must continue to honor and affirm our female wisdom and the sacredness of our bodies, even as we experience physical decline.

It is from our bodies that our Sagessence shines forth. When physical changes occur, we can deny them, or we can attend to the wisdom held in our bodies. We can look to the seasons of nature for understanding and integrate the truth of our oneness with all creation. Connecting our own cycles as women to those of Earth's cycles is a path to female wisdom, and fundamental to our sense and honor of the Divine. Envisioning a body-based relationship to spiritual renewal, we also can acknowledge the Divine similarities between our bodies and Earth. We will be amazed as we see the similarities between our regenerative powers and the regenerative power of nature.

After learning religious teachings reinforcing that my body was a mortal body of sin, I grew up in early life believing that I lived in a shameful container, not a precious body. It took many years for me to realize that the spiritual life is not one defined by religious scholars, but rather a knowing in the body that we are all one. A spirituality that celebrates the great web of interconnectedness among all creation and living things shows us how to honor both our Earth and our bodies.

As we embrace the concept that our bodies hold wisdom and sacredness, we can imagine possibilities of body prayer that involves movement and dance, singing and drumming, and playing other musical instruments. As with our creative practices, our spiritual practices can include drawing and sketching, painting, writing and poetry, photography, and gardening. We can also meditate by means of handwork, designing and crafting jewelry, and creating cards, quilts, and clothing.

We can learn to practice centering our energies daily in order to enter into intentional contemplation. Centering is sometimes referred to as "prayer of the heart."[20] When we quiet ourselves, descend into our depths, and focus on the center of who we are, we prepare to receive sacred wisdom. Centering is a process of achieving tranquility and inner stillness, with a listening manner. All of these possibilities can become spiritual practices and forms of meditation.

Of course, the spiritual path is enriched by the presence of others. Sacred circles are emerging across our country in which women gather to share their spiritual paths as soul companions for each other. Circles of women provide opportunities for growth, support, and community. Mutual respect for the wisdom of each person and commitment to accept diversity provides strength in the foundation of sacred circles of women gathering together. Strong support is prevalent among women as they share and discern their sacred paths. As women speak from their own truth, universality becomes apparent.

However we come to being spiritually energized, it is essential to know that we live from the heart of Divine mystery as we make new discoveries, and identify our passions, values, and truth. Rumi stated that God speaks to us through our loves, our most powerful inner feelings: "Love is the way messengers from the mystery tell us things."[21] We are called to believe what our listening ears hear from the depth of our Divine essence. We must understand that spiritual transformation is vital to the emergence of a maturing culture. In deepening our spiritual practices, we move forward in our lives, trusting in our own interconnectedness with Divine wisdom. Our families and the world will benefit from our personal experiences relative to accelerating shifts in the spiritual consciousness that is now emerging.

With Fire of Authenticity, meaning in aging is shaped in liberating images where we interpret the future. Our path of aging can be a path of grace, and rich and fertile with possibilities. Our future does not need to be a path of spiraling despair. It can manifest unexpected blessings and amazing achievements. It can be an era of immense satisfaction, as we become more of who we are as women of wisdom.

As we design our own unique blueprint with a Fire of Authenticity, we cannot help but soar a little higher. Sheila Huff, a fifty-four year old high school principal and adjunct university professor, participated as a member of Indiana's Women's Senior Olympic Basketball Team in Pittsburgh in 2005. Sheila shares her perspective:

> I feel like a very fine wine—getting better all the time.
> Years ago women didn't want to sweat.
> Today, it's a different ball game.
> Whatever I start I finish. I don't give up.
> It's just sending a bad message to me about myself—
> So, I see everything through.
> No broken promises anymore.[22]

No matter our age, whether fifty-four or ninety-four, and no matter what phase of life we are in, we will always find ourselves in a different ballgame. How will you, as a sage, play your authentic "ballgame"—your authentic game of life?

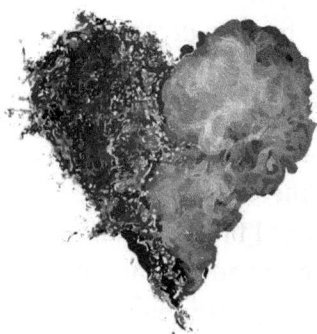

Chapter 3

The Fire of Passion

♥

Fire of Passion
invites us to live passionately in the moment,
to foster love, joy, wonder, and gratitude,
to deepen pleasures in our living, and
to make vital, life-affirming choices.

Living passionately brings inspiration to our days. No matter what circumstances or challenges we face in life, women in the second half of life can live with a *Fire of Passion*. It is with conscious intention that we can view life through a lens of wonder, joy, and gratitude. With increasing awareness, we have access to an abundance of ongoing pleasures in life. And from our wealth of wisdom, we can continue to make fulfilling, life-affirming choices.

The Fire of Passion path does not go unnoticed by others. It will influence many for good as we expand our sense of well-being and enhance our quality of life. This is our time to unveil passions. It is a time to live more consciously as we reclaim our capacity for love and joy, connect whole-heartedly to gratitude, and become attentive to forgotten places of wonder.

Enjoying pleasures in our daily life, and being clear about making life-giving choices will absolutely enhance our well-being.

Truly, we become more passionate about life as we become more aware of our impermanence. When we recognize a connection between impermanence and our amazing womanly potential, we sense an urgency to live fully every moment, in the present moment. When we contemplate naturally, we look long and lovingly at what is around us, and we take time to capture its uniqueness and depth. We learn the power of the ordinary in our lives, which moment by moment invites us to live with a never-ceasing sense of abundance.

Living Passionately

As we embody the Fire of Passion, we begin to live more fully in the present moment. We ponder with appreciation all life that is around us. When we recognize similarities with all living things and honor our interconnectedness, we cannot escape experiencing the awe and mystery of our existence in the cosmos. We become sensitive and awake to nature and its creative Divine energy that is ever-flowing in, around, and through us. Meister Eckhart, a 13th century mystic, professed, "God's ground is my ground and my ground is God's ground."[1] This is the "soil" wherein renewed passion is born.

Living mindfully is both a spiritual practice and a way of being in the world. Simply put, it is a way to restore inner peace and an inner knowing that we are part of the interwoven fabric of peace in the world. As we become

♥

aware of what is going on in our bodies, our feelings, thoughts, and emotions, we cannot help becoming more aware of all that is around us as well. Therefore, the art of mindfulness offers new refreshing ways to live in the present. It is learning to breathe slowly and fully as we become conscious to the moment. When we breathe consciously, we learn to recognize breath as a contact point with the air around us and then with all life that has been and will be on Earth. When we deepen this awareness, we open ourselves to wonder and passion for new self-discoveries.

When women in the second half of life live with a deep sense of interconnectedness with all life, there comes a deep respect for natural cycles from birth to death. We become increasingly aware of the precious gift of each day. There comes understanding that it is likely there is less time to live than time already lived. Embracing each moment of our lives with a Fire of Passion absolutely requires a depth of wisdom. The 14th Dalai Lama says, "Awareness of impermanence is encouraged, so that when it is coupled with appreciation of the enormous potential of our human existence, it will give us a sense of urgency that I must use every precious moment."[2] When we live with a sense of the immediacy of life, we can experience deeper joy and appreciation for the mysteries of life.

Fostering Love, Joy, Wonder, and Gratitude

The second half of life becomes a time to nourish love, joy, wonder, and gratitude. We develop keenness in recognizing more fully that divinity weaves in and through all of our relationships and experiences. All our relationships with each other, our god, and the cosmos are mediated through our bodies. Thus, our senses, emotions, and inspirations bring us feelings of love and help us live passionately. It is valuable for women to take time to consider each of these qualities and their significance for each of us individually.

Love. In *The Source of Miracles*, Kathleen McGowan discusses the immense and overwhelming task of defining love.[3] However, if we acquire a better understanding of the mysterious nature of love, we can understand more about how to experience it. Attempting to understand aspects of love is a wise effort, particularly in the Western culture where there is essentially no differentiation between the vast expressions of "love." We toss the term around in our conversations from loving our partners to loving pizza, all in the same breath. It wasn't until I began to differentiate meanings of love through the Gnostic teachings that I was able to begin unscrambling my personal encounters with love and expressions of love.

Even by briefly glimpsing the Gnostic teachings of love and finding six definitions, you may be startled by an "aha" moment. First, *agape* love is the word most often translated in the gospels as spiritual love or Divine love. It is the experience of love that involves the joy we experience with another, and in a kind and compassionate world. McGowan calls it "the purest form of spiritual expression." It is unconditional and considered the "highest love." *Philia* is the love of true companions, of friends, and love between close siblings. It is relative to mortal love in comparison with the spiritual nature of agape. *Charis* is love that is defined by grace and devotion. It is a love that bridges heaven and earth; a love for god as well as for our earthly mother and father. *Eunoia* inspires deep compassion and commitment in service to the world. This is where our love for charity in our community dwells, integrating our inspired hearts and our stimulated minds into active service. *Storge* is a pure love that is full of tenderness and deep caring. It is an innocent, playful, and sweet expression. It is how we express love for children, or describe the love we feel for our pets. *Eros* defines romantic love as well as sacred sexual love. It is an abstruse celebration in which souls come together in union of physical bodies.

Even in considering these six types of love, we are still left with great capacity for depths of mysterious loving encounters. These short explanations of love from the ancient Gnostic teachings begin to rouse interest to discover deeper meaning of the word "love" that we use so freely today in our culture. While a solution to a better world is to love more, the questions remains, "How do we broaden our experiences of love?"

Indeed, a challenge for us is to broaden our capacity to love. Experiencing love differently in relationships is not about controlling or possessing others. And it is not about permitting ourselves to be controlled or possessed. Women in the second half of life are seeking new depths of love, different than previously experienced or expressed. For many women, such love may not yet have been discovered, or even well-defined. In the poem, "Story of Intimacy," new notions of a deep loving encounter may be roused:

> I yearn
> to live a story of intimacy,
> beyond my youth,
> beyond mid-life,

beyond society's meaning.
I desire to be deeply known,
yet fear being known
both at the same time.
It is my profound need,
like food to eat,
water to drink,
air to breathe.

I reach for waiting arms
of deep intimacy.
At times I touch its sweetness
while thinking,
I may keep secrets my own.
Yet, the voice of intimacy
asks me to share
tender stories of my heart,
of my mind,
of my soul,
share them with another
imperfect human being—

Allow another to discover
what moves me, inspires me,
drives me, hurts me,
makes me smile and sigh,
what I am running toward
and running from,
what I whisper to the gods at night,
and what silent, impish enemies
still reside deep within,
what wildness I harbor

and what wonderful dreams
still wait deep in my heart.

What is your story?
Do you have a deep need
to be known—
to be discovered,
and re-discovered
over and over in a lifetime?
If you do, take my hand
and don't go away—
I promise to not turn from you
and perhaps, dear one,
together we will discover
a new story of intimacy.[4]

It is rare for women and men to find partners who love in this manner. For those fortunate enough to experience this kind of love, life is lived as if there are two bodies and one soul. Also, if we love with our hearts open, we may even weave in and out of relationships—coming together and letting go— in ways that show honor and respect, while never forgetting the depth that was shared. In this way, we carry others lovingly in our hearts, while acknowledging the reality that two individuals are truly moving on with their lives.

One of the sage's foremost and grandest responsibilities is cultivating a deeper capacity to love well. Oriah captures my point here: "I allow myself to imagine that each moment in which we love well by simply being all of who we are and being fully present allows us to give back something essential to the Sacred Mystery that sustains all life."[5] Living as instruments of love, we absolutely must learn to *love well*. Again, Oriah beautifully explains:

> I want to make love to the world by the way I live in it, by the way I am with myself and others every day. So I seek to increase my ability to be with the truth in each moment, to be with what I know, the sweet and the bitter. I want to stay aware of the vastness of what I do not know.

For each of us to define how to live in this way is truly important. There are vast ways to love well and radiate love, extending beyond family contexts into the world. It may be through our presence, our attention and support, communication on many levels, or through our work and service, to name a few. Not only is loving well essential, but it is the best we give that emulates living our Sagessence.

Deeper tenderness and fulfillment can be attained in meaningful relationships. I witnessed this deepening in my parents' relationship, as conveyed in the poem "Grand Love:"

> She was 92.
> Her beloved was 88.
> They warmed me
> like few lovers have.
> Their tenderness,
> respect
> and gratitude
> prevailed throughout
> their late season days.
> And only like
> old sweethearts can,

The Fire of Passion

they always discovered
satisfying ways
to express steadfast,
tender love;
to share gems
of intimacy
that come with time,
and grace hearts
with fulfillment.

Growing older
day by day,
they beheld each other
with grand love,
a mystery
nothing could deter.
Although years claimed
their harsh mark
in many unfriendly,
unkind ways,
gazing into each other's
wise eyes,
holding each other's
feeble hands,
truly dismissed
any naive notion
that seasoned love
could possibly belong
to man and woman
of their youth.

The world yearns
for what they shared,
like writing
I love you
on plaid, flannel backs
in the night,
stroking white hair
with gnarled fingers,
blowing kisses
through windowpanes,
eyes twinkling
with mischievous,
ancient laughter.
Their endearment
was not for taking
but to be witnessed
as they continued
their art of forgiveness,
their joy of being
dearly loved.

They knew their breath
was precious life,
and did not allow
a loving moment
to escape
their few fragile days.
They engaged
soulful pleasures,
ever imbued
by simple delights.
And, like old lovers

with new eyes,
they gazed tenderly
under drooping lids
into windows
of each other's
dear soul,
treasuring grand love—
their legacy
of love's sweet mystery.[6]

A way to view expanding our experience of love is to consider the immensely mystical experience of "falling in love" and, relative to this, essentially falling in love with life. Matthew Fox suggests that,

In fact, we could fall in love with a galaxy every day and, since there are one trillion of them, bequeath many quite virginal on our deathbed. Or we could fall in love with a star, of which there are 200 billion in our galaxy alone.[7]

Fox continues to encourage us to look to that which surrounds us and is so obvious—to behold nature for infinite opportunities to fall in love. He suggests that we consider the natural world, "a species of wildflower, of which there are at least 10,000 on this planet. Or a species of bird, of fish, of tree, or plant."[8] Of course, we can also fall in love with another human being. Essentially, we can imagine expansively, looking for ways to be in love with life. We can open ourselves to the multitude of joyous possibilities to fall in love every day.

Joy. Joy emulates from wonder and awe, and fosters a sense of gratitude. It is scarce in many women's lives. Yet it is critical to our spiritual, emotional, and physical well-being. It makes life worth living. Consciously answering the question "What brings me joy?" actually holds the key to bringing more joy, pleasure, and ease into our lives. It helps us connect with what nurtures and renews our spirits, and feeds our souls. Many women struggle with this question because they experience little joy in their lives. Joy has been displaced by frustration, stress, illness, perpetual activities, busyness, as well as constant and rigid routines.

Debrena Jackson Gandy shared what many women in her seminars have identified as sources of joy.[9] Women shared that joy can be experienced by singing, bathing, reading a good novel, receiving long hugs, napping, or relaxing in front of a fireplace with a favorite drink. Enjoying stimulating conversations, making love, getting a massage, or savoring a delicious dish prepared by someone else were also joyous. Creative activities such as writing, poetry, sewing, quilting, painting, playing musical instruments, and many other creative expressions also provide women with enjoyment.

Although joy does not evolve exactly the same way as laughter, the two are certainly many times connected. All of us can certainly remember many times in our past when we found ourselves in a synergistic enjoyment of belly laughter with other women. It emerges spontaneously in women's comradery in the midst of sharing that is candid, real, and honest. Laughter arises in the midst of crazy, embarrassing stories of triumph. Hilarity unfolds. We may not be able to catch our breaths, our bellies may ache, and our tears spill over. Endorphins flow, we experience joy, and our sense of well-being is enhanced. Most of the time, we cannot retell the course of humorous outbursts with the same level of intensity. That is okay. Although, our bodies and spirits have experienced the great benefit of laughter.

Humor is fun, and it can also extend our lifetime. It is medicinal and healing. Studies have shown that women who infuse themselves with laughter have had miraculous remissions from disease, or even healed. Jean Shinoda Bolen states that healing humor acknowledges and makes light of difficulties that unite us rather than divide us.[10] Whenever there is an absence of affection in humor, it does not leave us with a sense of well-being. Humor that is an outlet for hostility, or puts down or diminishes others, is an act of attempted superiority. We benefit from humor that creates a sense of freedom and celebration, and that fosters joy in communion with others.

Could it be that for the sage, laughter is an expression of the victory over matters that could have broken our spirits? Is it the medicine that protects us from bitterness? Is laughter the vocal applause over something that happened or didn't happen that we come to accept and make the best of its situation? Even when living in difficult or confining circumstances, we can be enlivened by joy. Lily, age ninety-eight, shared with me her joy of watching and identifying birds that gathered around a birdfeeder outside her window at a local nursing facility. She also enjoyed frequent personal conversations with young female employees. Lily said, "Those young women need someone to listen to their stories and problems about their families. They have a lot on their minds with all the work they have to do around here, and then go home to more. Sometimes, I can give them a little help and encouragement. Sometimes, we can even have a laugh or two."

Elene, an eighty-seven-year-old resident in a rehabilitation center, enthusiastically anticipated the nightly visitation of a resident cat that came and snuggled on her feet at bedtime. She was mystified why the cat chose her. However, she truly looked forward to the lights being turned out and then joyously anticipated her friend's arrival in her room. Elene missed having pets and found renewed joy befriending the tabby cat that lived there.

Maria, in her late seventies, shared with me the joy that the art of painting had brought to her heart. When she was in her late sixties, her husband passed away. With more time available to reflect, she remembered when she was a child and loved to "paint" mud on old shingles that had blown off the barn. She bought acrylic paints and supplies and decided to teach herself how to paint landscapes. Maria found that her hours from waking in the morning to retiring for the evening disappeared as she painted fervently. She discovered that she could not learn fast enough, so she hired an artist to teach her how to develop her skills. Soon, Maria sold some of her paintings just to help with her supply costs, she said. When I met Maria, she had lost her vision. Her love of painting became a welcomed memory rather than a daily passionate activity. Although she grieved that she could no longer see to paint, she was extraordinarily grateful that she had seized her moments—*carpe diem!*

We might ask, "Why do so many people settle for so little joy when there is so much wonder and awe everywhere?" Meister Eckhart shared related thoughts:

It is because they live lives of entertainment of the outer person alone and never bother to explore the inner and then the innermost person. The outer person enjoys the loaf of bread, a glass of wine, and a slice of meat merely as bread, wine, and meat. The inner person also enjoys bread, wine, and meat but in that enjoyment does not taste merely the food but also the gift that the food is. Thus, the inner person nourishes a sense of gratitude and even wonder at the gift that the ecstasies of creation bless us with.[11]

The sage lives consciously with loving intention. There is wisdom in living with deep affection and intense emotion. Whether it is through an intimate relationship with a lover, the thrill of simple pleasures of life, or giving our energy and time to social causes, we can expand our experiences of love. By learning to love well, we access a wisdom that also holds the powerful potential to increase our capacity for joy, gratitude, and wonder.

Wonder. One of the most intriguing life experiences is the simple act of basking in wonder. One of my favorite pastimes is to sit on ocean-side rocks and imagine how they all arrived in their places. I wonder where the beach glass came from and from where did the driftwood originate? What happened in the lives of the creatures that inhabited the seashells? What vast life resides beneath the waves that roll in and out from the shore?

You may explore various activities to sharpen your awareness of wonders that are in your midst each moment. You may become intrigued with the mysteries of life that you simply may not have previously explored. Simple moments that may have previously eluded your attention may now cause you to ponder and muse. Regardless of the circumstances of your life, when you look for and discover things that are awe-inspiring, you continue to attract moments of inspiration.

Wonder carries an element of wisdom that is innate in each of us and that we have carried from childhood. To understand this, take time to observe children in their play and their discovery of the world. We, too, were designed and wired for a sense of wonder. For many women, the overlay of daily demands obscures our natural characteristic of experiencing wonder. Not only can we experience wonder and delight by honing our awareness of nature and creation generally, we can evoke wonder with what we, as women, create and birth in the second half of life. Wonder is deeply connected to the depths of our creativity and passion.

When we reconnect with our sense of wonder, there comes a renewed appreciation for the splendor of life. I express my deep appreciation and awe in the following poem:

Magnificence of Life

I have tasted
magnificence of life
for which
I have not words...
rendered voiceless,
wordless—

Wordless,
like an unborn child
not knowing
how to possibly describe
marvel of It's existence,
a spectacular gem

♥

nestled in a corner
of Its mysterious
womb of life.

Simply,
voiceless,
wordless

Ah, wise
seasoned sage,
savor magnificence
of your life
for which
you have not words.

Speechless,
like a newborn child
not knowing
how to possibly express
marvel of your existence,
yet understand that
your essence is
your gem,
your wealth.

Simply,
voiceless,
wordless

Savor this moment,
honor yourself,
and the magnificence

of your precious life
in this world.[12]

Gratitude. As we become more conscious of many phenomenal blessings experienced every day, we strengthen our ability to live with a sense of gratitude. We not only need to internalize gratitude, but express it as well. We could describe experiencing and expressing gratitude as what Debrena Jackson Gandy describes as a concept of "conscious gratefulness."[13] Gandy believes that as we learn to deepen gratitude and appreciation from the situations and circumstances that come our way, we can contribute to a *culture of gratitude*. In general, our culture is one that is ungrateful. Have we been spoiled by technology and creature comforts? Are we luxuriating in waste and excess? Do we take things for granted and feel entitled to material gain?

Rhonda Byrne, in *The Magic*, takes the necessity for gratitude to a deeper level. She states, "Gratitude operates through a Universal Law that governs your whole life."[14] She explains that relative to the "law of attraction," which regulates all energy in the Universe, *like attracts like*. With the law of attraction, when we give thanks, we receive more for which to give thanks. Simply stated, without gratitude, we cannot receive what we desire in life.

In elder years, many simply seem ungrateful by the process of aging and challenges they face physically, financially, and socially. It is not uncommon to hear comments such as, "The Golden Years aren't so golden." It helps to remind ourselves that opportunities to be grateful come to us in various events, situations, shapes, and packages. It may not be apparent at first, but may become more visible as time goes on. Nonetheless, it is essential to keep foremost in our consciousness that the more we are grateful, the more we *see* with grateful eyes.

Practicing gratitude can assist you in identifying greater pleasures. Being grateful indeed helps you keep the events of your life in perspective. Sages cultivate a practice of gratefulness that helps develop a shift in our personal attitudes that, in turn, potentially shifts the cultural perspective.

Deepening Pleasures

With a Fire of Passion, there is deepening of pleasures by hearing, touching, seeing, smelling, and tasting in ways not previously experienced. Greater delight can be experienced when we consciously savor colors, shapes, and textures. You may be moved to awe simply by hearing the wind beneath the wings of geese in flight, feeling misty rain on your face, or watching sunsets often interwoven with rich colors and dynamically changing cloud formations. Pleasures can be enhanced, by inhaling the sweet fragrance of flowers or savoring the sweet tastes of various wines. You may recognize an inner longing to be in touch with life, as well as to touch and be touched.

As we age, physical touching and emotional connections become more important. Although research shows that we remain sexually alive throughout life, many women may not choose to remain sexually active.[15] However, honoring feelings and exploring a variety of options for experiencing bodily pleasures remains important. A woman's body is a channel for experiencing pleasure. If we are tense or stressed, sensations of pleasure do not move through our bodies readily. As sages, we can become aware of more fully opening our bodies to the flow of energy and experiences of pleasure.

Life's pleasures are possible and available to us regardless of what day it is, how old we are, or the amount of money we may have or do not have. Pleasures bring delight, a sense of well-being, and a greater quality of life. As aging women, pleasures that enhance our sense of well-being and our quality of life may be simple pleasures that we will no longer take for granted.

As I reflect on a past journal entry, I clearly see two women's perspectives—my mother's as well as mine—relative to simple pleasures. This is what I experienced on the morning of my mother's ninetieth birthday, and mirrors pleasure in unpretentious moments:

It takes my breath away momentarily when I realize how many times I have remaining to see my mother again. Possibly, I could count them on one hand— maybe two hands—since I only see her typically twice a year. This morning, I held her hand, and ran my fingers across the frail skin that draped over the structure of her other delicate hand. She smiled with quiet appreciation. I feel lucky to be with her again.

I sat on the edge of her bed as we chatted about her day. It was then that I first noticed her eyelashes are now very thin wisps of white down. Gone are the light brown lashes that could once be extended with conservative applications of mascara. I noticed how her fingers beautifully tapered to such lovely nails, although half painted with clear polish this morning. Crazy, but I couldn't help but try to fathom momentarily all that her small hands have done in ninety years.

With the oxygen tubing trailing her every step, I

helped Mom to the bathroom. As she began her usual morning routine, I could not help but notice how heavily she breathed as her chest heaved up and down. I realized breathing is a body's task that I, for one, have personally taken for granted all too often.

As I assisted Mom in getting ready for her bath, her clothes fell to the floor, piece by piece, and revealed her diminishing and yet beautiful petite porcelain body—still with lovely feminine curves. Her small breasts draped towards her rounded belly. Slight ripples now replace the once smooth skin of her still lovely-shaped legs. With so much dignity, she insisted on washing her genitalia. I splashed water for her as she rubbed the liquid soap gently with her hands. She then turned and eased herself down on her hands and knees into the bubble bath she asked I prepare for her. As she slowly swiveled her small body into the water, she moaned with contentment, followed by a sigh of seeming relief. No doubt, her sounds were grateful expressions of the utterly comforting caress of the warm bathwater. Her almond-shaped eyes looked up into my eyes, and her thin lips turned into a smile as she asked, 'What are we going to do for lunch today?'

I handed her towel to her opened wide, then reached for an arm to help her step out of the most glorious of daily routines. As I patted the back of her legs dry—the part that she could not reach—she stood gazing out the east window of the bathroom. Once again, after fifty-eight years of mornings on this farm place, she took a moment to savor the beauty of the rolling pasture hills now waiting for spring. We both stood quietly in the moment—she in awe of the morning and I in awe of her.

Mom interrupted her gaze and reached for her

underwear. She took my hand to steady herself as she stepped one foot and then the other into the leg openings. My heart ached observing her struggle to pull her panties up over her tummy. I quietly responded to her request to help as she slipped her arms into her bra. I gently tucked her elongated breasts into cups much too perky for her mature shape. I wondered how bras could be designed better for ninety-year-old breasts. As I connected the middle hook in the back of her bra, she thanked me, and reached for her lotion.

I stood quietly with my heart full of love and waited as she pulled her robe around her small fragrant body. As I reached for the doorknob, she looked up into my face and smiled sweetly. I can hardly believe this was the morning of Mom's ninetieth birthday. Where has it all gone? How did our time slip away so quickly?[16]

As women become older, it is necessary to embrace life with greater care and with deeper respect than ever before. Deepening pleasures certainly includes being mindful of our self-care. As we embrace opportunities to deepen life pleasures, there comes peaceful realization that we are participating in a magnificent plan of ongoing abundance. We then truly embody the Fire of Passion and become more hospitable toward our aging.

Making Life-Affirming Choices

By embracing our Fire of Passion, we learn to honor and respect the earth and all inhabitants of the earth. We learn to live simply and to move away from accumulating and cluttering our lives with complexity. Our capacity to live with a sense of harmony and balance is awakened. The power of the ordinary in our lives becomes meaningful. Our self-care contributes not only to the quality of our life, but also influences our families. When we accept the processes of change that are inherent in our living, changes that result from the choices we make become more easily accepted and honored.

To sustain the Fire of Passion, sages continuously make choices from a self-supportive vantage point while focusing on decisions they consider life-affirming for others. This approach is paramount for aging women and positively influences families and others. In this regard, there is an inspiring story told by Pamela Peeke, M.D. about Edith Odoms, a retired schoolteacher from Walla Walla, Washington.

Edith was confined to a wheelchair after falling and breaking her hip. Regardless of the challenges she faced, she was determined to heal her body and become independently mobile again. On Edith's ninetieth birthday, she asked her daughter if she thought she could benefit from a program called "Body for Life."[17] Her daughter was supportive, and Edith committed to succeeding at her new health endeavor. She began lifting weights three times a week from her wheelchair. Improvement was slow; however, Edith was excited about each incremental improvement. A few weeks later, Edith said she was ready to get out of her wheelchair; and in her words, "One day, I just got up out of it—slowly, but I did it." She began to walk for minutes a day, walking and resting repeatedly. By two months, Edith was walking one mile in twenty-three minutes. Soon thereafter, she walked three miles a day. Her physical health as well as her mental outlook continued to improve.

At ninety-five-years-old, Edith was taking martial arts classes, senior fitness classes, and strength training three times a week. She ascended and descended stairs on her own, got up from chairs, got in and out of her bathtub as well as cars. Edith reported that her diet was healthy, too—plenty of fresh fruits and vegetables and lean protein. She said. "I gave myself the gift of a whole, healthy body. I tell myself if I slow down, there's another wheelchair waiting for me. My goal is to go on and never give up."

Edith's story helps us realize the potential we have to make life-affirming choices, as well as to imagine far-reaching influences our choices may have. I doubt that Edith would ever have thought her story would be included in a book or women's group seminars, such as my "Living Our Sagessence" seminar, so that untold numbers of women could learn from her courage. Decisions we make every day as sages have the same exponential possibilities.

In the second half of life, our decisions become more influential. When choices are made from the center of our authenticity and with a sense of self-compassion, we can believe that what is downright good for us is downright good for everyone else. Choices reflect regard for self as well as for others, as we become exemplary sage models for other women. And no matter how crazy our choices may seem to others, where else can an answer come from to the question, "Who can I ask to tell me what I came to make happen in this world?" The answer must come from the depths of our own wise spirit. After all, who else could possibly be the wiser for our choices?

In *The Search for Signs of Intelligent Life in the Universe,*

❦

Jane Wagner addresses possible underpinnings for choices women make:

> You're thinkin': How does a person know if they're crazy or not? Well, sometimes you don't know. Sometimes you can go through life suspecting you are but never really knowing for sure. Sometimes you know for sure 'cause you got so many people tellin' you you're crazy and it's your word against everyone else's.[18]

Our choices may seem absurd on the surface; however, they may hold depths that will change the course of our lives and provide deeper fulfillment. Many times, decisions may not even make sense to us, but our spirits insist that we embark on a new direction that we are called to trust as our path unfolds.

A few years ago, Nancy, a retired Episcopal priest, came to my office for her annual follow-up appointment. She said that she was finishing up business and moving to Mexico. Surprised, I inquired about her decision. Her story unfolded. She had recently traveled with a friend to a village in Mexico. Her friend knew a group of women in the village and wanted to return to visit them. While there, Nancy became acquainted with a circle of strong women who welcomed her, offering their loving hospitality and friendship. Three days into her stay, she made the decision to buy a home and move to Mexico. With a huge smile of anticipation the afternoon of our conversation, Nancy showed me her photo—there she was lying in the bathtub of her colorful adobe home with a big smile and a glass of wine in her hand. A tall woman, her criteria was that if she could fit into the tub, she would buy the house. Offering herself a toast, she decided to do just that!

Nancy returned to Washington and told her family of her decision. They were a close-knit family, and she had chosen to live nearby during her retirement. Her son and his family conceded to her decision. However, they wondered how she would be able to easily visit her aging sister in San Diego. She replied that it was a mere nine-hour bus ride to San Diego. Confidently, and not without grieving, she proceeded to plan her future. Nancy said that for the first few nights after making her decision, she cried herself to sleep anticipating leaving behind her fifteen-year-old granddaughter, in particular. However, she believed that the best gift to herself on her eightieth birthday was to live a life she had dreamt of and never chosen. She also believed that her personal life-affirming choice would provide an example for her granddaughter to make courageous choices for her own life. Furthermore, she knew her granddaughter would delight in visiting her in Mexico.

Often life-affirming choices that women make on their own behalf require others to adapt or adjust relative to the effects their choices may have on them. At times, the choices made prove to be life-giving for others. The most profound example that I have personally experienced relative to such an effect resulted from my mother's choices made while hospitalized a month before her death. An excerpt from my journal reflects mutually beneficial choices she made in ministering to her family while hospitalized and in a dire state of health:

Life is so fragile, and death so tough. Mom continues to struggle to live. Every breath is such an effort! What dualism—this body and spirit.

Most of the grandkids have now come to see her. Yesterday, she asked that a chaplain come to her bedside to pray for her and the family. There were hours of delay—apparently there were other emergencies requiring prayer, so no chaplain was available. As evening approached, I wondered why we really needed a chaplain, someone we don't know and doesn't know us, to create a sacred time together. So we all gathered around in Mom's room, circled her bed holding hands. Immediately, *she* started to pray for each and every one of *us*, and for her grandchildren yet to be born, for generations to come. Amazing. We had an awesome time singing favorite songs she requested, and sharing from our hearts.

Dad and I got settled in for bed afterward, and then around 11:00 p.m. I felt an urge to return to the hospital. When I arrived, Mom was in crisis. I called for her nurse; the respiratory team was then called. Throughout the night, they worked diligently to keep her breathing. Her wishes for 'no resuscitation' have been documented clearly. Yet when doctors recommended that she be put on a respirator in intensive care for a procedure to clear her lungs, Dad trumped her wishes and gave his approval. I was clearly ambivalent about the wisdom of his choice. Nonetheless, the medical staff diligently moved forward.

Today, the respirator was withdrawn. The procedure relieved Mom's breathing distress immensely. In preparing to return to Seattle tonight, I felt a real urgency to have time alone with her. I hate knowing that our time together on Earth is now so limited and we have few moments alone, just the two of us. I asked her nurse for uninterrupted time alone with her before I left the hospital tonight. As I entered the room, I was stunned to see her face was like fine porcelain, softly glowing with an amazing glorious peachy hue. Her anguish and agitation had dissipated; deep crevices carved by endless pain and struggle had been replaced with subtleness and peace. I can't remember when she has breathed with such ease. My heart leapt as she smiled and gestured for me to sit next to her on the bed. In those moments together, I experienced the greatest gift imaginable.

We shared our love and appreciation for each other. I told her she would always be my angel and she said I would be hers. I wept, and she feebly reached for the Kleenex and compassionately wiped my tears with her gentle, trembling hands. She passionately loved me with motherly tenderness, and showed acceptance that I have longed for. In those sweet moments, she explained how proud she was of the woman I have become. God knows my heart has struggled for years, as we seemed to grow further apart the more my life path diverged from the world she has known. Yet as she beheld me and I her, there was a deep womanly knowing and respect, beyond all differences, and our hearts were imprinted with each other's love. In those moments her actions healed deep wounds of separation as she stroked my face and consecrated my life with loving words, "May God glorify your life, my dear daughter, and all that you do." This was her benediction.

Death was gracious to wait, and Dad was wise to listen to death's instruction. What more should I desire? Nothing. The past is the past. I take her loving consecration with me, and hope there is just one more time together before this woman who birthed me and has enduringly loved me, surrenders her life here and continues on her wondrous way.[19]

❤

As a woman who lives consciously in the moment, you cannot help but become more acutely aware of the mysteries of life that emerge from living passionately. Trusting there will be enduring gifts revealed, look long and lovingly at what is around you in which there may be riches emerging that you cannot even predict. Wouldn't it be wonderful if you were left dazzled, reveling with gratitude for all the unpredictable blessings and graces that came your way? Even this is a conscious life-affirming choice that you can make.

As we reflect on our Fire of Passion, we would do well to remember that we belong to a supreme reality greater than ourselves. In this larger context, we rediscover the mystery within which everything is endowed with purpose and meaning. As we embrace mysteries inherent in the Fire of Passion, we can celebrate with this teaching in mind, knowing that our passionate living is our choice and will emanate far beyond our personal lives. All of life is a gift and blessing from the Divine and is truly at the heart of our sacred journey.

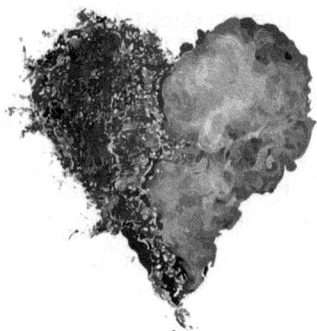

Chapter 4

The Fire of Compassion

♥

Fire of Compassion
stirs us to practice loving kindness,
to live in the flow of loss, grief and change,
to graciously give and receive care,
and to move through life transitions confidently.

The path of the woman sage strengthens as she embraces the *Fire of Compassion*. In reality, all creation is immersed with compassion. It is the ultimate blessing we give to ourselves and to others. The Fire of Compassion is a way of living and walking through life with loving kindness. Matthew Fox speaks of compassion in this way: "It is the way we treat all there is in life—our selves, our bodies, our imaginations and dreams, our neighbors, our enemies, our air, our water, our earth, our animals, our death, our space and our time. Compassion is a spirituality as if creation mattered. It is treating all creation as holy and as divine . . . which is what it is."[1] The capacity to experience our interconnectedness includes honoring joy and sorrow, gain and loss, as we experience relationships with others. In loving others, we deepen love for ourselves. Indeed, these are essential elements in living compassionately.

We gain deeper understanding of compassion when we grasp that grace is also an integral part of the Fire of Compassion. Fox provides further clarification:

Compassion is not about pity or feeling sorry for others. It is born of shared interdependence, an intuition of and sense of awe for the wondrous fact that we all live and swim in one primordial divine womb, we live in fetal waters of cosmic grace![2]

In our culture where aging is not revered, there is a deficit of compassion for older people. Compassion toward aging citizens is absolutely a primary need. We can begin to shift this reality by learning well the benefits of self-compassion on many levels. Women, regardless of age, can effect change for the greater good by both giving and receiving compassion. Then, as we consider our shared interdependence, we can strive to become inspiring examples who do not make judgments based on age, sex, title, conduct, manner of dress, height, weight, skin color, religious affiliation, political beliefs, or family structures. We open ourselves to relationships that are absent from all-knowing, possessive, or demanding viewpoints. And we approach situations and others with loving curiosity and patience.

There is an imperative need for women sage leaders to let others choose and pursue their own way of life, from a foundation of their own conception of highest good. We cannot know what others should or should not be choosing in their life paths. As sages, we view our loved ones as capable and competent of making good choices, with wise counsel as needed. Yet, of course, we must be proactive if choices others make are self-destructive or potentially harmful. In that case, we can create opportunities to be inspiring: offering encouragement and guidance for them to achieve their own greatness.

As you deepen in self-compassion and trust your authentic nature, you may notice a generosity of spirit emerge. This generosity of spirit allows others to live authentically as well. People become more genuine, trusting, and willing to stand in their own truth.

Practicing Loving Kindness

Kindness is integral to the practice of compassion. As sages open their hearts to practice compassion, they must learn to be kind to themselves so they can truly be kind to others. I recently saw a plaque in a gift store that stated, "Remember, there is no such thing as a small act of kindness. Every act creates a ripple with no logical end." Wouldn't it be mind-boggling to fully understand the expanding effects kindness has on our own lives, let alone the lives of others?

Kindness blossoms when we consider ourselves as well as others, and when the two sides are in harmony. It is part of our original human nature and typically is a resource that women can readily access. We all have moments when the openness and beauty of our kindness shines. When we lose connection with this tenderness, we must remember that it can be reawakened. In meditation, compassionate kindness can be breaths away, with a quieted mind and with an open, loving, and understanding heart.

Buddhist teachings describe compassion as "the quivering

of the heart in the face of pain, and the capacity to see our struggles with *kindly eyes*."[3] The source of disharmony in many relationships, families, communities, and around the globe is a lack of awareness, or a lack of knowledge, relative to given situations. Personally, we may be blind to our own states of denial, envy, anxiety, pain, or underlying grief. Unfortunately, layers of ignorance and trauma can obscure our ability to be compassionate. When we identify our own lack of foresight, we can begin to open our hearts and extend kindness.

We need kindness to help us be tender with our difficulties. When we transform bitterness or despair with acts of kindness, we gain insight and strength to pass through difficulties without lashing out or increasing pain and anguish. We need it when children or grandchildren experience difficulties, when we face illness, or when we confront other challenges such as divorce or death. We can become vulnerable when things go awry. At these times, everyone involved can benefit from acts of loving kindness. Compassion calls us forth to listen intently—with encouragement, love, and respect.

In a sage leadership paradigm, there are various areas of concern to consider in expanding cultural perspectives relative to kindness. Kindness is a behavior marked by ethical considerations. It reflects a pleasant disposition and genuine concern for others. It is a virtue that is recognized as a value in many cultures and religions. It encompasses greater awareness and openness for inclusivity. To stimulate your thinking about ways to expand your views, and thereby cultural views, relative to compassion, considerations relative to family, marriage and re-marriage, and divorce are targeted here for your contemplation.

Family. Family is an abstract concept involving the perceived quality of worthiness and respectability that affects a group of related people. Although "family" is a concept, it truly is a living, breathing organism. It is comprised of generations of members as well as those connected to the group through birth and marriage. In our culture, our communities highly value the relationship between honor and the family. Conduct of family members reflects upon family honor and ways the family perceives itself and is perceived by others. Behaviors include social conduct, religious practice, eating and dress habits, possessions, educations, lifestyles, and livelihoods.

In our culture, we perceive family as a core institution. Our social identity depends largely on our family. Therefore, for the most part, it is important to consider or fulfill expectations of our family and culture to experience a sense of belonging. In some families, maintaining family honor is considered more important than autonomy, authenticity, individual freedom, or personal achievement. Many times a family may attempt to overpower the actions or beliefs of an individual. At worst, they may disregard or shun a member. On the other hand, a theme that is common within many traditions is the integral practice of respecting elders.

A sage leader will honor the tradition of family, and yet kindly and prudently consider variance from the norm of the traditional family model. Shifts in our views of family will expand definitions of family and family dynamics. In addition to what we have experienced in traditional families, society will consider gay and lesbian families, single-parent families, blended families, and adopted families as inclusively typical in a new definition of "family." A compelling question is, "How can I expand my definition of family with a sense of kind-heartedness?" This is a compassionate question.

As we expand our definitions in this society, daughters, sons, and grandchildren of the family will respectfully honor their elders in ways that see them as keepers of wisdom and valued informants. They will understand that once an individual has lived life for several years, they have earned a position of tribute and should be shown such regard. As well, elders will uphold their family members as capable, and with high regard and belief in their best potential.

Marriage. How can our kind acts affect views of marriage relative to moral diversity? Marriage typically provides security—by law, by social convention, by ideas of respectability. It has been a norm consistent with earlier generations. However, great personal disharmony can be created by marriage. Many times, early marriages result in divorce, or bring lives of discontent or even misery.

Numerous things have changed in the post-technological era we now live in. The institution of marriage, as it was initially established, is no longer necessary as such. People live together now without being married. More and more women are becoming financially established and have resourceful careers. They are also now making choices about whether they will or will not birth children, and they are making choices about whether or not to marry if indeed they do have children. Single women may choose to adopt and/or have biological children. Lesbian marriages are becoming more prevalent.

In an evolving world, it is excellent counsel to encourage our children and grandchildren to discover and come to intimately know their own personal preferences, values, priorities, hopes, and dreams. Maturity in knowing oneself well provides a wise infrastructure to explore many relationships and life options before making decisions that could possibly be limiting otherwise. Considering the extent of this type of personal homework, so to speak, there is no longer a need to hurry into marital relationships and contracts.

As the ideology of marriage shifts, sages envision spiritual partnerships or marriages between equals based on core conscious choices for mutual support, love, respect, and honor of the highest aspects of each other's spiritual unfolding and *best version of self*. This is a radical shift from experiencing marriage as a union grounded in cultural expectations.

Daphne Kingma imagined new and illumined forms of marriage, with sacred vows and a dedicated commitment to explore the bounds of conscious partnerships. Whether through deep psychological work, spiritual practices, or tantric sexuality, new possibilities provide gateways to higher transcendence. Kingma challenges us to turn a "spiritual somersault" and experience our relationships in ways that are more the truth of love and kindness. She explains:

I believe that we are being invited by Love itself to have our relationships become more and more about love—the energy of love, the power of love, the meltdown of love, the passion and compassion, union and communion of great love.[4]

This is very different from marriages based on material benefits, attempting to resolve emotional issues, procreating, maintaining social structures, or personal ego. It is revitalizing to envision marriage as simply based on genuine loving kindness.

Considering the prevalence of divorce, savvy married women will keep a pulse on the infrastructure of their marriage. It is important to bear in mind that circumstances of divorce and considerations of re-marriage also provide opportunities to re-envision aspects of marriage that are not life-giving, as well as re-visiting the qualities of marriage that remain desirable. Also, the complexities of re-marriage are vast—blended families, non-traditional families, prior relationships that remain a part of one's life, and other experiences and memories that have integrated into our bones. Regardless, it is truly a missed opportunity if we do not give ourselves the gift of viewing our relationships with sincere gratitude for all that has been good, and with willingness to re-define ourselves in ways that we can truly become better people as well.

Divorce. NationMaster.com reported in February 2010 that 50 percent of marriages in the United States end in divorce. Although divorce typically challenges our very foundation, women initiate the largest percentage of divorces. According to data published by American Academy of Matrimonial Lawyers in June 2013, people over the age of fifty are ending their marriages more frequently than ever before. Cathy Meyer, divorce support expert, reported data found in a 2014 nationally representative study by the American Association of Retired Persons (AARP) that shows women initiate two-thirds of divorces and even a higher percentage of separations (divorcesupport.about.com).

Although women typically turn every stone over in an attempt to save their marriages, they are becoming less tolerant of relationships that are less than emotionally, intellectually, spiritually, or sexually satisfying. They are willing to take risks to move on with intentions to create more of what they desire in life. Although postulations point to a high possibility that a woman may be disappointed again in a subsequent relationship or will experience guilt to varying degrees relative to leaving her husband, she courageously chooses to move on into the unknown. With this in mind, how do we hold the tension of divorce with new depths of kindness?

At the turn of the third millennium, Debbie Ford spoke of the "spiritual divorce."[5] With kind eyes, one may begin to see all the events preceding the divorce as leading to the exact place they are supposed to be. An individual's perception shifts allowing one to see the former spouse respectfully. Then, with as much grace as possible, the individual uncouples from past relationships and moves forward with gratitude and anticipation. Thus, divorce can be an experience of greater gain than loss. The experience of divorce from a marriage union can be viewed as an opportunity for deeper spiritual transformation and greater self-expression. It can serve as a beloved friend that seeks to lead a woman into unexplored thoughts, beliefs, and territories.

Typically, women in this culture are affected in some way or another by family, marriage, and divorce. These areas can have a vital impact on our lives, and many times the effects can be more profound in various ways as we grow older. This is particularly true since we are such relational beings. A fundamental undergirding in our relationships is to deepen in our ability to love and express kindness. Of course, here again the leading principle is that we must learn self-love and self-kindness. This most fundamental thing has to happen within us first. Loving ourselves is absolutely necessary and foundational to being able to truly love others. The fact of the matter is that you cannot love, or extend kindness and compassion, to any greater extent than that which you offer to yourself. Absolutely, any increase in self-love, self-intimacy, self-compassion, self-acceptance, or self-forgiveness will immediately increase your ability to extend love, intimacy, compassion, acceptance, and forgiveness to others. Treat yourself with love, regard, and respect. Be true to yourself. You will deepen your gifts of kindness to the world as you experience the alchemical shift that emerges from deepening in these ways.

Living Through Loss, Grief, and Change

The second half of a woman's life may be viewed as an important and rewarding developmental era in which she becomes more authentic. She becomes more courageous, more thoughtful, and introspective. She is better prepared to develop psychologically and spiritually than during any previous time in her life. However, there are many losses experienced as we age that challenge even this foundation of maturity. We grieve for our youth, our strong bodies, our sense of being needed, our independence, and our tattered dreams and ideals that we see no way of regaining. There may be losses resulting from deaths of spouses, partners, children, and friends. These are all experiences and closures that become more meaningful when we gain wisdom from the Fire of Compassion.

Our greatest opportunities to practice compassion emerge by embracing loss, mourning, and darkness as natural processes of living that are shared in oneness with all creation and cycles of existence. We endure losses throughout our lives. Some are small, and we hardly notice them. Yet there comes a time for most of us when losses become more frequent, overlapping, and irreplaceable. We learn how intrinsic pain and suffering are to love. The experience of loss affects both who we are and how we care. We must learn how to mourn all kinds of losses and gain comfort by acknowledging natural, shared rhythms with all of Divine's transformations.

As sages learn to better understand loss and grief, they come to realize there are many variations of grieving. Nonetheless, grief follows a general path. It takes us through a period of numbness or shock, into a time of disconnection and possible confusion, and on to new ways of connecting with self and others. We may circle many times through the stages of grief, and not by a linear process. Ultimately, as women, we not only recover parts of ourselves, but we find energy to relate in different and enriching ways.

In tending to our healing and grief, there are positive ways to support our process. It is helpful to connect with a reverent listener, a companion who can hold our emotions and pain. Second, if we can believe in love in the midst of our loss, we can also acknowledge a loving Divinity within our own being. It is also essential that we anticipate that we will lose and find our sense of self again, yet with greater capacities. Creating rituals that are significant to express the meaning of a loss enables women to mourn with the support of intimate women's circles. As women staying close to the parables of nature—that resonate clearly to life, death, and hope of vital new beginnings—we intuit our losses in the mystery of all life.

Managing inevitable difficulties with realistic optimism requires befriending our inevitable losses. In many ways, loss takes us into darkness. An analogy is to consider the wonderful mystery that our bodies are filled with darkness. Our heart works just fine in the dark. Our liver, our intestines, and our brain are all beautiful and harmonious working parts of our magnificent body going about its everyday business, day and night, completely in the dark. How awesome. Imagining the beauty of the inside of the female body cannot help but fill us with wonder, gratitude, and praise for what amazing things can happen in the darkness of our own physical temples.

Matthew Fox succinctly describes the journey of embracing the darkness of loss, which is relative to all who embark on a spiritual path: ". . . we will know God as we know ourselves. We will journey into God as we journey into ourselves. If we can face the darkness within, we can face the darkness that is God."[6] As we courageously embrace our darkness and learn to live through difficult times, we gain resolve by learning to let go and let be. Fox states that Meister Eckhart's description of "letting go and letting be" translates to entering into nothingness, and requires a process of emptying ourselves so that the Divine can move in and through us.

In letting go and letting be we learn to cope with two of the greatest spiritual challenges of aging: loss and change. It is a place where sages not only rely on their wisdom, but also rely on the weaving of the Divine's energy throughout the process. It is well to understand that "letting go" cleanses the conscience, inflames the heart, and awakens the spirit in yet a different way. As aging progresses, events in our lives that require us to change become more prevalent. We typically attempt to retain control of life circumstances such as vitality, health, finances, mobility, and relationships. This is reflected in "Letting Go," a poem from *Fire in the Well*:

> As evening came in her latter years,
> her heart wrangled with letting go—
> letting go of possessions,
> ideals of health, infinite independence,
> and life itself.
>
> Letting go of dreams
> incomplete, unfinished,
> that escaped from her fragile reality—
> replacing desires with mustered hope
> of just one more day doing what she loved.
>
> She nestled in the comfort and safety
> of her rocking chair in a quiet living room,
> wisely surrendering
> to honest gratefulness
> to fulfillment in reminiscing joy.
>
> With soft smiles on her thin lips,
> she gazed tenderly into faces of those she loved
> while struggling to let go,
> still wanting to hold on,
> yet surrendering to the evening of her life.[7]

Independence becomes a higher premium as we recognize that society has a negative attitude toward dependency. There are more experiences of loss in many aspects of our lives, regardless of how hard we try to keep our lives in order. Actually, it is in our later decades that we will make more changes than at any other period in our lives. These changes inevitably involve loss. Paradoxically, losses are especially hard because we have devoted most of our days to acquiring the very things that begin to go away.[8] We may lose our friends, our spouse or partner, children, our home, a job, and possibly financial security. Possibly our most profound loss is actually our grieving for the ultimate loss of self.

Lavina, a seventy-eight-year-old woman, wrote about her experience of returning to the place where she and her deceased husband had lived, raised their family, and made a living. The process of letting go and letting be is deeply sensed in her poem, "Memories":

> The old home place is changed now-a-days,
> And dear ones who lived there are gone.
> Someone else now tills and waters the fields,
> And cares for the garden and lawn.
>
> My memories I'll store gently away,
> In a place known just to myself,
> There they will quietly rest in repose,
> Like toys standing long on a shelf.
>
> New doors have opened, new friends I have made,
> New ways have come over the years.
> I'm a new person—ah yes, I have changed,
> Though sometimes with shedding of tears.

The time has sped by, I'm older by far,
And I've learned much over the years,
As not spending time with sighs and regrets,
Instead, scattering joy and good cheer.

It's not through getting but giving we grow,
Not hoarding but sharing we gain.
Wealth and position don't matter so much,
It's that God is with me on this plain.[9]

Lavina beautifully conveys the repose and peace she had gained in letting go. Her wisdom is apparent in the way she relates to her history with harmonious acceptance of the fluidity of life. A sagacious woman, she reframes loss into more meaningful ways of being, yet no doubt with struggle in reaching her conclusions. In sharing what she learned over the years, it is clear that Lavina realigned her priorities and then followed through with discipline to create her best life. She clearly understood that opportunities arise out of new beginnings that evolve out of endings, which are integral to the life journey.

In our later years, we are increasingly faced with difficult circumstances that can only be resolved by letting go of our need to understand or reach reconciliation with them. We may fight change to the bitter end. Ultimately, either we choose to let go and let be, or we risk becoming stagnant. In the process of letting go, emptying, and letting be, we may gain peace and wisdom trusting the evolution of God's love and work in our lives and in the design of the cosmos.

There are times when we may feel lost in the turbulence as our lives abruptly change due to unexpected circumstances that are inconsistent with our intentions. We may become confused, uncertain, and sometimes overwhelmed. These are times when we might look to other women to learn from their wisdom and to gain hope. Understanding and discernment are what we may need. This longing is reflected in the poem, "I Want to Know":

> I want to know
> what sustains you
> from the inside out
> when your gut twists,
> rolls and wrenches
> from unmistakable taste
> of sour injustice,
> or when love turns its back,
> or when your dad dies.
>
> I really want to know
> what gives you hope,
> what gives you joy
> when all else crumbles
> down around your socks,
> as if your life were leftovers
> disintegrating to crumbs
> swept off your table
> right before your eyes.
>
> What keeps you from
> running for cover,
> hiding under the eaves
> of your otherwise
> good-looking life,

when claps of thunder
or heavy, humid smell
of an impending storm
looms in your bones?

Tell me about what
ignites juicy desire
in your soul once again,
what strikes a flame that
bursts forth your *yeses,*
your passionate songs,
blazes with inspiration,
helps you hit high C . . .
with your heart unzipped.

What makes you tilt
your gleaming face and
throw happy hands
up to the radiant sun,
topless and barefoot—
even if the neighbors,
your dearest friends,
or perhaps your kids,
think you've turned crazy?

I just want to know.[10]

We may reach a new level of comfort and assurance as we
surrender to wisdom, and hope that greater possibilities
will manifest if we remain open in the bends and turns of
our sacred journey.

Releasing what has previously been integral to our lives

purifies us and cleanses us, allowing our hearts to awaken to other possibilities. It is in our courageous willingness to open to the unknown whereby the Divine continuously enters and enlivens us. It is in letting go that we see Divinity in and behind all things. This is a powerful view of spirituality in aging. Herein is hope to bear fruit and birth newness again, which is especially comforting as we live through perpetual challenges.

In *Gift from the Sea*, Anne Morrow Lindbergh writes about the art of "shedding."[11] The shedding she speaks of seems analogous to the process of letting go, for it feels like darkness and death. But it can also be the liberation by which we become at last completely ourselves. How does one then enter into the art of shedding with grace and confidence? Is it simply by trusting there are no endings without new beginnings?

A few years ago, my husband and I had the opportunity to vacation in the New England states. One afternoon while driving in the Catskill Mountains to enjoy the colors of autumn, we were prompted to stop along the roadside and simply take in the beauty of the moment. It was a perfect opportunity to witness shedding relative to the lovely descent of fall leaves. I sat on a rock wall and scrawled the poem, "A Day to Let Go," which depicts the ongoing cycles of nature's autumn endings and pending gestation of new beginnings:

> Today is a day
> to let go
> of all that has been.
> In extraordinary moments,
> with this one as witness,

leaves simply let go
of all their life has
been in seasons past.

From voluptuous buds
alive with vibrancy
of succulent green,
sensuous yellow
to hot fiery orange
then majestic red,
they now relinquish
to a graceful descent:

Turning away,
floating, twirling,
flirtatiously dancing,
gliding up,
drifting down,
veined edges to the heavens,
gracefully suspended,
without breath at all.

In these mysterious
final moments—
is this what living
has prepared us for:
a grand surrender of
letting go into the
soft, cool lap of Gaia,
our holy, sacred retreat?

Today is a day
I dare ask my question,
What else do I
desire of me?
Listening intently,
a soft echo rises
in the cool, damp,
mountain breeze.

It is the simple sigh
of the awed witness—
yes, also suspended
like without breath.
I wait in the leaves
for an answer, breathing,
What else do I
desire of me?[12]

When we encounter darkness and nothingness resulting from our experiences of loss, the Fire of Compassion helps us realize that silence and emptying, letting go and letting be, and pain and suffering experienced during times of loss are integral parts of living. They are also integral to our spiritual journey. However, we can trust the time will come when we will emerge from loss, from our pain and sorrow.

As we age, we begin to realize that the many kinds of darkness we encounter can be opportunities to gain a deeper capacity for love and joy. As we move through the darkness, in the end the same spiritual challenges exist: to know that the Divine is somehow present even when it is not apparent, to see impasse as a call to new hope and vision, and to deepen our capacity for love. We can envision transitions as new opportunities for life. In reframing our context of darkness, we can come to view darkness as a path to greater hope. Like the caterpillar in winter, hidden within a tightly closed cocoon from which it will emerge one spring day as a butterfly, so also are we slowly transformed in the darkness. This is a profound metaphor for renewed hope.

Hope is essential to every human life. A disturbing aspect of aging is when we assume the future is devoid of hope. Hopelessness may result from experiences of despair, grief, and fear that are part of our humanity. Each of these is a natural response to loss and vulnerability typically associated with cultural views of aging. However, such experiences may prompt us to make changes in ways we live, and in ways we choose to renew our souls and deepen our faith.

The process of inevitable endings and beginnings offers opportunities to gain greater wisdom and personal wholeness. You can be transformed by personal loss and by losses of others. This progressive development occurs through, not apart from, what you cherish and desire in your life. Therefore, in changing your context of loss and grief, you can alter what typically has been viewed with negative connotations. The dark night of the soul is indeed a special occasion for a sacred birth and opportunity, provided you let the darkness be darkness at least for a while, and trust that light will enter again.

Giving and Receiving Care

Giving care is a tough and earthy practice. It raises

fundamental spiritual issues for women as they enter the second half of life. Each of us who lives long enough will know it in many forms. We care for children, parents, friends, a spouse or partner, and/or brothers and sisters. We ourselves may experience conditions that leave us weak and dependent on others for basic tasks. We touch love in its fullness as we move through these experiences.

A commitment to caring is a living practice that takes into account all that is happening to us in the present moment. It is not unusual to find contradictory emotions within us when giving or receiving care. A core issue is what we do with what we feel. The more we are able to accept a range of feelings in ourselves, the more responsive and receptive we can be to others.

Many times, women are powerless in the face of suffering, loss, and pain. We feel sad and helpless. It is excruciating to stand by, unable to do anything. The ability to do something, almost anything, helps us deal with the pain. Sometimes there is literally nothing we can do, except be present. I remember tenderly the extraordinarily difficult hours that followed the tragic vehicle accident that took my brother's life at the age of thirty-five. While my family waited at the hospital in shock and disbelief, hours passed as my brother was given every opportunity to survive. A friend of mine and my husband's arrived at the intensive care waiting room and asked if we would like him to join our family and us. Paul Welter didn't know my brother, Wayne, nor his wife or children. He didn't know my mother, father, or other immediate family members. What he did know is that we needed support, love, and compassion. He knew we would need a glass of water, here and there, and a shoulder to cry on. Paul didn't know what to say to ease the pain of that tragedy. However, I will never forget his loving presence through those painful hours. He never left our side until we left the hospital after my brother passed away.

Our friend demonstrated the practice of "withness" whereby he simply committed to being present with us as we struggled. He remained with us without knowing what to say or what to do. I wrote about the commitment to "being present in the moment" with those we deeply care about, as reflected in the poem, "Heartland of Our Souls":

> I will stay with you in this place
> no matter what you need
> or how long it takes
> for gain of strength
> to move on again.
> I will remain as your companion,
> whiling away time,
> seeking calm solace,
> feeding on leftovers in stubbles,
> bedding in tall reeds of cool rivers.
>
> There is no need to go anywhere,
> nor return
> to my place called home.
> I wait on one leg,
> then another,
> in the hospitality of hidden blinds,
> patiently keeping loving watch
> with uninterrupted gaze,
> attending compassionately,
> guarding your peace of heart.

Of course, that is until . . .
in an instinctual moment,
like crimson-crowned cranes,
majestic wings spanned wide,
bodies stretched long and lean,
we fly toward fields flourishing
with abundant harvests,
beyond the beyond,
heavens welcoming our soar
into another intuitive unknown.

Yes, you can count on me.
I will stay with you until,
like crimson-crowned cranes
called to dances
in other fertile fields,
either you . . .
or I . . .
take flight from this place
to another land—
the heartland of our souls.[13]

The dilemma of caring is that it asks us not only to hold onto, take care of, empathize, and suffer with those we love, but it also asks us to step back from and let go of them. Many times, our attachment to a preferred outcome precipitates our own suffering. However, we can stand only so much contact with pain and suffering. We need refreshing experiences. Remembering that our own health and well-being may be at stake can lead us to take time away for essential self-care.

Nonetheless, we can experience many of life's most

priceless moments in situations of care. One of the most sustaining gifts of caring—the feeling of joy—comes from this fulfillment of relatedness. Joy occurs, even in the midst of grief and pain, when we find ourselves genuinely joined to another. A good relationship is something highly valued by both the one giving and the one receiving care. It allows room for greater intimacy. As we are filled by the caring relationship in this way, our capacity for compassion deepens.

Caring for others is a valuable opportunity to increase self-empathy by enabling us to direct our sense of understanding and responsibility toward ourselves, as well as toward others. Balancing our needs is essential. Denying our needs does not reduce another's suffering; it only limits our ability to support another. We need to keep a separate sense of self.

A spirituality of care relative to our changing times calls us all to create more effective forms of care for the future. A combination of increased life expectancies and women's increased participation in careers has created a crisis for continuing care and support. We have contributed to this situation by assigning women the role as primary caregivers without providing them appropriate and supportive resources such as respite care, employee leave for family care, and affordable home healthcare. These are critical social issues to be addressed, as are issues of justice for the elderly.

Generally, most people do not eagerly anticipate the task of caring for another person in physical and/or mental decline. Many deny that the need is coming. Avoiding preparation can place any one of us in an *unprepared* caregiver role with a moment's notice. Wise preparation is necessary to avoid such "baptism by fire." We all need to assume that we are likely to be a caregiver someday in some capacity. The reality is that the number of unpaid family caregivers is growing exponentially every year. Therefore, the smart sage considers the spiritual aspects as well as the logistical decisions of such sacred work that will no doubt move us, as well as the one in need, into and through unknown transitions.

Honoring Transitions

Aging becomes a mosaic of transitions and passages. The sage understands that tremendous change can happen in life every day. Yet life goes on flowing; nothing is frozen in time. The past is always closed; the future always remains open. In between the past and the future is the present, moments in which there can be trembling and shaking. The sage anticipates change while understanding it is inevitable in transitions as we move through a passage from an ending to a new beginning. She holds herself with honor and respect, and gains greater sensitivity throughout the process.

Some transitions result from our own choices. Others come from circumstances beyond our control. Regardless, the process takes us from closures and relinquishments, through emptiness and darkness, to fresh opportunities and new life. This movement reminds us of the cyclical nature of all of life: the pattern of the seasons, the waxing and waning of the moon, the ebb and flow of the tides. Women's lives include many cycles of stability followed by periods of transition. Transition is integral to any transformation.

Navigating your way in and through transformation is typically very difficult. However, you can focus on navigating with poise and dignity, attempting courageously to make transitions confidently. Although endings that lead to transformational beginnings are essential to your process, it is natural to cling to the familiar and fear the unknown. Transitions take you through a continuous course of losing and finding a new identity. Circumstances change you. Who you thought you were, you discover you are not. Roles are always in flux. Even your behaviors within roles are always in flux. Not only do situations change you, your values may change because of situations. When you realize your role as mother, grandmother, wife, partner, employee, or businesswoman (to name a few) shifts in the midst of change, you may question your identity and your place in the world. You may begin to wonder, "What is real, and how real am I?"

Our deep questions may arise from a place of feeling that we have arrived in a wilderness—an uninhabited place or inhospitable region. We may know for sure that we would not have chosen to go there, sensing such an emotional place with disfavor. There may be perplexity, loneliness, and uncertainty in our waiting, as I conveyed in the poem, "Wilderness":

> I feel nothing.
> After years of feeling so many things,
> I touch the mirror and wonder,
> *Who am I becoming?*
> Strangely, I feel silence.

I walk along the sea's shore
and gaze into summer's night.
I sit in my den and listen for god.
I share love and practice kindness.
How can I not feel beyond this quiet?

Have I been banished from
imaginations, dreams, and passion
that previously inspirited my life?
Can I not conjure up some thing
that entreats my heart not to sleep?

Lowering lids and graying temples
remind me of lessening time as
I wonder if this is sane—
a freakish cleansing of my spirit
before the last sprint of my journey?

Is this . . . *wilderness*?
Am I engulfed in a Divine ambush
that begs me to rest in the backwoods
of my soul and wait for the
truest of my nature to quicken?

Does this wilderness know
what I will leave behind . . .
what I will claim as my own?
Does this wilderness really
know my name?[14]

Although many times transitions result from significant
life-changing events, there are times that profound, or

maybe even subtle, invitations to change begin to stir in a woman's soul. Sensing that something is ending and the time has come to let go may arrive in a slow, intuitive, internal shift, or may result from a significant initiation of new awareness. Similar to birth contractions that come to separate us from the safety of the mother's womb, or separate us from our fetal child, a hidden timing begins to stir bringing a sense of readiness for the new. Our focus begins to shift, and we are no longer able to live our old identity.

Transitions are a time for sages to discern the calling from within. In an attempt to reach clarity, they gather information, talk with friends, seek support, and consider options. It is fertile time that allows space for the work of our creative and imaginative selves. These powers may work slowly and quietly at a deep level of the self. We clearly sense an inner prompting, yet we may need to wait for clarity.

Endings and beginnings both require periods of transition and, hopefully, fresh new life prevails. Resolution is not always swift and straight. We move forward and frequently circle back, although we never actually return in the same way. As we listen, we begin to know what we must do. Often we are aware that clarity has been reached when we begin to tell others what we intend to do.

Our lives include many cycles of stability followed by periods of transition. Change is not simply a moment in our existence. It is a pattern in our lives, similar to the rhythms of nature, as reflected in an excerpt from my poem, "Great Masters":

As surely as . . .

brown eight-eyed orb weavers
float another silk line
to the October winds,
And
little purple and white crocus
hardily push through winter's snow
as promise of new life,

Great blue heron will arrive
at woodland nesting grounds
spring after spring—
And
I will pause a summertime eve
recalling bittersweet
and tender farewells in winter.[15]

Transitions may lead us to move on to a new path or may result in staying in place as we discover newfound ways of continuing. Outcomes can be novel and unexpected. Nonetheless, transitions provide opportunities for women to live out the truth of their discernment. It is a time to trust courage and hope, which are two gifts of the Fire of Compassion.

In my audiology career, I interacted primarily with individuals over age fifty. There were many rich opportunities to learn from patients about their attitudes, opinions, strategies, lifestyles, and stories of endings and beginnings. Their lives encompassed varied circumstances: from baby boomers at last realizing they are indeed aging, to many who were in their ninth and even tenth decades and whose lives reflected the challenges and triumphs of aging.

A few years ago, one of my patients scheduled an appointment for a seemingly insignificant reason. It was promptly clear to me that his thirty-minute appointment was more accurately five minutes for service-related reasons and twenty-five minutes to share what had recently transpired in his life.

There was a slight twinkle in his eyes when I asked how he was now that his wife, Mary, had passed. He confidently assured me that he was doing quite well. There was a sense of peace and joy on his face that I had not seen over the four years he had been my patient. A nudge in my heart prompted me to wonder if he may have fallen in love since his fifteen years of care-giving for Mary had concluded. He loved Mary dearly and had cared for her compassionately. Often, I had seen tears in his loving eyes as he spoke of her. However, today there was something different about him.

Marvin continued to share that Mary's decision to die was made one night the previous fall. He said she looked lovingly across the table during dinner and said, "This is my last meal." Mary had previously contemplated that starvation would be her friend whenever she decided her quality of life would no longer bring either one of them further joy. That particular night marked the conclusion of her contemplation. Her husband vowed to respect her wish.

There was never another shared meal. Mary kept her vow, and Marvin kept his promise to support her. Although hospice became involved, she was resolved in her decision that it was time to leave. Three weeks later, almost exactly to the day, Mary died. In her final days, she encouraged her beloved husband to get his "show on the road." Marvin laughed joyfully, yet sad tears moistened his eyes. He told me she was a wonderful woman whom he had been privileged to be with for fifty-two years. At the end, she encouraged him to get on with his life, and to find a friend to enjoy. She encouraged him to take a good look in the mirror because she was sure he would like what he saw.

After Mary's death, Marvin moved. He left the assistive care facility where they had lived, and rented a delightful apartment of his own. He unpacked belongings that had been in storage for years, and began to enjoy the romantic company of a friend. With a renewed twinkle in his eyes, he exclaimed, "Bring on the tuxedo and the symphony!" He laughed as he shared that he was now eating three meals a day that he cooked himself, ate on his own fine china and sterling silver unpacked from storage, and enjoyed classical music more than ever before. He had renewed his commitment to good health practices and felt he was "seventy-eight going on sixty."

Marvin no doubt grieved for Mary during previous years as they faced the challenges of her declining health. With a compassionate heart, Mary helped her spouse embrace the ensuing chapter of his life. As he left my office that day, he shared that Mary had taught him that happiness is found in enjoying every moment fully. Second, she helped him realize the profundity of giving lovingly to causes one believes in, as well as the importance of attending to dreams.

Our conversation that afternoon was enough to substantiate Mary's apparent philosophy of continuing possibilities, opportunities, and contributions. She had learned to let go and let be, to encourage her husband to create newness of life, to embrace each moment passionately before and after her death. She also lived her commitment to die with dignity and on her own terms.

Quite frankly, Mary Hood Evans was a sage activist. She and her husband were active supporters in filing the 1990 Death with Dignity Initiative 119 in Washington State, which was marginally defeated. Mary's courageous end-of-life decision reflected her passionate belief in personal choice relative to death. She transitioned before the Death with Dignity Initiative 1000 passed in Washington State's election in November 2008. In a recent conversation, Mary's husband fondly shared reflections of their political efforts and their continued commitment to this core value.

Many women internalize society's images of aging and have conventional assumptions about how the second half of life is expected to evolve. As previously noted, our culture has typically regarded aging as a process of moving toward a peak of optimal living, then proceeding to a downward slope of diminishing abilities, effectiveness, and experiences. With this model, aging becomes a fall from independence and power, unlike Mary's choices.

Closures that lead to transformation are essential to our process and ultimately to the process of others. There can be no rebirths without completions. Some part of us believes this, yet many times, we are drawn to that which remains familiar. For certain, a woman is no longer the same person after important life changes. She bids farewell to one sense of self without knowing what she will be like in the future. Regardless of how difficult or unexpected the progression, we can embrace our unknowing and honor the impending change even before we are clear how life will unfold.

Although, even as sages, we cannot predict what parts of

our sense of self may require revision, we can rely on prior experiences to know that we will survive any transition and change that may arise. We will continue to further live with life experiences of sorrow and confusion, embrace moments of joy and ecstasy, encounter success and failure, and undergo betrayal or miracles of grace. Life will always continue to give us opportunities to learn wise teachings from gains and losses. This is especially possible as we live with a spirit of gratitude and appreciation for all that has been, all that is, and all that will be.

It is well to remember that our most holy work as a sage emerges from the Fire of Compassion. This path manifests the fruit of the spiritual journey and reveals Divinity within us and in others. When we grasp this understanding, we can internalize that all of life is a gift. All life is a blessing from the Divine and is at the heart of our sacred journey of aging. Divinity is in the innermost part of each one of us; we cannot live in separateness. Deepening understanding of these spiritual aspects can enrich our aging immensely and provide support for challenges we will no doubt face.

The Fire of Compassion offers many ways to engage in compassionate living. Compassion is indeed the first blessing we receive, and the ultimate blessing we give to ourselves and to others. Most profoundly, compassion is spirituality in its maturity. And it is fundamental for profound fulfillment in our life journey.

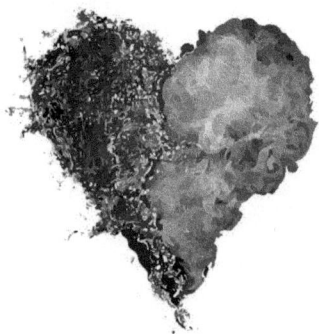

Chapter 5

The Fire of Vision

♥

Fire of Vision
calls us to create a living legacy
that supports greater good,
to manifest deeper fulfillment,
to impart a wise, mentoring spirit,
and to honor intergenerational connectedness.

Imperative to the *Fire of Vision* is the call for women to embody their visions as they create their living legacy. In changing how we view aging, we realize the importance of continuing to focus on fulfilling our dreams, pursuing meaningful projects, and making valuable contributions. When we awaken our Fire of Vision, one of the most valuable investments we can make for current and future generations is to impart our wise mentoring spirit. Furthermore, as we comprehend the magnificent interconnectedness of generations and all living things, we honor our lives as absolutely essential in the history of the Universe and its continuous unfolding. This is conveyed in the poem, "My Child," which I wrote for my daughter:

You, my daughter,
carry in your mind
my spirit of seeking,
in your bones
my spirit of wisdom,
in your heart
my spirit of love.

You
came to me, called
by passion of my soul
longing for more,
further than myself,
in gifting the world
beyond my life.

You
carry me past
my future into yours,
expanding afar
my grandest imagination
with your own
exquisite spirit.

You
take me with you
into many tomorrows,
transcending into
that ever-continuing
sacred thread of
Wisdom's legacy.[1]

Integral to this path is recognizing that what we generate, as women in the second half of life, becomes a legacy of the self. What more powerful role can the aging population have than to accept this challenge?

As we engage life with our Fire of Vision, we must trust our own visions. We can learn to quiet our minds and hearts to become attuned to receiving knowledge and guidance. We can go on vision quests, which involve days of solitude, fasting and prayer, in pursuit of guidance from Divine intelligence. We can connect with our spiritual visions during times of deep intuition, through night dreams and day dreams, and during expanded states of consciousness. Through meditation and self-hypnosis, we can open ourselves to visions. Some visions come in full color, so to speak, with detail and clarity. Other visions appear in images and unfold over time. The fact of the matter is that throughout time human survival has depended on human visions.

Many people in our Western culture are immersed in technology and materialism. They have lost sight of even the possibility of being channels for visions. With their heads figuratively separated from their bodies, they have drifted into chaos and faded away from the palatable intelligence of the Universe.

As we begin to grasp the intelligence of the Universe, we begin to see that there is an "evolutionary potential" that seems to be growing. Barbara Marx Hubbard emphasizes, "There have to be members of the planet who wake up and guide this power for the sake of life. It is awakening in millions of us now that something new is needed . . . . It has been my experience that most people waking up to this fact are women over fifty."[2] We are called to wake up as women sage leaders to the powerful potential we have to recognize our visions and access deep wisdom to illuminate the way during this dynamic time in history.

Creating a Living Legacy

Our society typically thinks of "legacy" as a gift of property, especially personal property or money, by will or by bequest. It is considered anything handed down from the past, as from an ancestor or predecessor. However, is it not what we live now that really matters? Is it not the positive influence we can create every day? What if we intentionally imparted our passion for justice, our property, money, values, ideals, love, and our wisdom right now?

Seasoned women are called to blaze a new path in creating living legacies as sages. As women fully living our Sagessence, we cannot take for granted the gift of having the opportunity to live an extended lifetime compared to previous generations. Longer life is now our unique, untapped resource, gift, and creative challenge. This challenge calls us to not squander our abilities, talents, or gifts, but to celebrate them and uphold them to be resources in achieving ongoing transformation for our society.

As women change the societal context of how we view aging ourselves, we become aware of a starting point to value the action we can take to intentionally live our own legacy. Older women become more self-assured and willing to take gambles in order to follow their priorities. At different points along the path of aging, women are likely to stand up for justice—personal and social—take a stand on issues, and make life choices not previously believed to be achievable.

In the second half of life, there comes an inner prompting to share our talents and resources to make a difference beyond our own private lives, which extends out into the world. As women sage leaders, we seriously consider ways we can contribute to our families, communities, and broader concerns. We determine what is important and create room in our lives for what is significant relative to our passions, such as family, children, friends, various causes, and contributions to our local and global communities. Acts of generosity may include sharing our possessions, money, knowledge, and emotional support. We gain meaning, purpose, and fulfillment when we find opportunities to make positive changes, believing that every good and kind act contributes to the better welfare of the world. Our choices and contributions matter and do have widespread affects.

As women unveil their personal living legacies, many will also rise to challenge the worldview that they inherited. In these times of rapid change in the world, we are challenged to change whether we intend to change or not. Our viewpoints may evolve to reflect major developments in our civilization. As we experience new ways—what we believe is real, then our ways of thinking, opinions, and worldviews typically change. This includes what we think is real relative to matters of God, the economy, technology, and the planet. This concept also involves what we value and how we treat our beloved ones. It includes what we think is real about our life priorities, lifestyles, ways we spend our time and money, and changes in our livelihoods. As women assume leadership roles, they are taking matters that were once considered personal issues—matters privately discussed—and bringing them into public view.

With a Fire of Vision, women effectively become agents of transformation working toward a living legacy of a more caring and compassionate society. Collectively, we have enormous abilities to impact the health of society and our environment. Many women clearly demonstrate that there are rich and diverse opportunities to take action for positive change. Issues to consider include how to give back to the planet, how to work for justice and peace, and how to handle political issues more collaboratively. Women can channel their interests to relieve suffering and confront injustice. We can participate in humanitarian relief organizations such as Habitat for Humanity. Another organization, PeaceWomen Across the Globe, aims to increase the visibility of women promoting peace all over the world.

Our next generation, women in their forties, are making huge benevolent differences in their communities. Jennifer and her partner, who both work in the private sector, have keen understandings of the power of women in business. They have participated in an interesting and ingenious opportunity to help others help themselves through Kiva. This is a nonprofit organization with a mission to connect people through lending. For several years, they have recirculated loans through Kiva for women in third-world countries to establish their businesses. Leveraging the internet and a worldwide network of microfinance institutions, Kiva lets individuals lend as little as $25 to help create opportunities around the world. When a loan is paid back to the donor, the donor can then elect to recirculate the loan back to another Kiva recipient. This is an opportunity to alleviate poverty.

I am impressed with continued efforts of other women in their mid-years connecting benevolently with their visions. Kristen, a project manager for a Fortune 500 company based in the Northwestern US, is influential in including that company in making dreams come true for children with life-threatening illnesses through Make a Wish Foundation. She also extends her compassionate endeavors in her advocacy work to transform the lives of rescue pets, through actively supporting the mission of Homeward Pet, a nonprofit organization with a mission to give homeless animals a second chance through rescue, shelter, and adoption.

Nina, who has a nursing career, runs and raises funds for benevolent causes. A marathon, half-marathon, and triathlon runner, she runs to promote the vision of organizations she believes in. Nina runs "so the world can see, hear, feel, accept, and embrace" causes from cancer research to promoting peace. Having spent a segment of her career as an intensive care nurse at Madigan Army Medical Center, she participates annually in "Race for a Soldier" to help fund post-traumatic stress treatment for women and men returning home from military service.

There is a plethora of other ways to become involved in transformative action. We can become involved in promoting alternative approaches to healthcare. Of course, there are numerous ways for women to be active in volunteer work, including hospitals, daycare centers, schools, community help centers, and county and state parks. We believe that our actions can make a difference as we find ways to support children's education and their well-being. Our concerns about violence and the abuse of women and children can also lead us to find ways to take a firm stand and keep a hard line for greater social transformation.

Annie, a woman in her mid-fifties, shared that she never expected that she would be working with traumatized victims of human trafficking. Although Annie does not see herself as a leader, she says, "I am a servant at heart." Her vision to help in this regard was inspired by her daughter's story about working with trafficked individuals in Thailand. This brave, bright, and determined young woman, along with two other young women, desired to educate locally about this global issue. Their goal to educate quickly turned into a nonprofit organization serving their local community, with far-reaching influence.

In my conversation with Annie, she said, "This love makes me brave, strong, and passionate. As we fight these seemingly overwhelming battles, I carry within me a bright flame of hope and joy. I still find it surprising to hear myself say that I love doing this work. I have the blessing of seeing the awesome changes taking place in the lives we have the honor of touching." Annie's story and her daughter's story reflect two generations of living legacies that are creating a wide swath for the greater good of women and society.

Women sages focus on discerning their visions and attending to the work that supports bringing them into reality. As we consider radical ways that we can create new possibilities for our visions to take form, sometimes what we need to do is begin by simply trusting the raw images. Consequently, we gain confidence in subsequent manifestations that potentially can emerge from them. We learn to rely on and stay true to the inherent wisdom that unfolds. Whatever we choose to do is always our choice; however, it is entirely possible that the guidance that comes through visions could have significant value.

The Fire of Vision

❦

Margaret Wheatley encourages us to keep faith in our visions. To emphasize, she quotes Rainer Maria Rilke:

> You must give birth to your images.
> They are the future waiting to be born.
> Fear not the strangeness you feel.
> The future must enter you
> long before it happens.
> Just wait for the birth,
> For the hour of new clarity.[3]

Therefore, in contributing to societal change, it is important to attend to visions that emerge from your consciousness and be willing to bring them into reality with form. Recognize your inner gifts; understand your mission. It is your responsibility to know what these are. Do not hesitate to share them. There is no time in our lives that provides richer opportunities to take action than in the second half of life. Now, take a few moments to consider ideas in areas that you may find inspiring as you consider creating your living legacy.

Children. The greatest action we can take may just result from guiding our children and grandchildren, our nieces and nephews, and even neighboring children. This awesome responsibility calls us to higher standards as family and community members. To consciously encourage each child's uniqueness, self-awareness, and contributions with greater acknowledgement and respect is essential. We must be patient with children, and very mindful not to hinder the development of their intelligence. When the child starts inquiring, her/his own miracles start happening. We must learn how to best inspire each child to satisfy their curiosity and refrain from giving ready-made answers to questions. Offer situations and challenges to sharpen intelligence, and to build self-trust and self-confidence. Otherwise, there will always be a need for outer guidance and a lack in their ability to trust their own potential and competence.

Encouraging our children and grandchildren to make their own decisions confidently, as soon as they are able, supports a new foundation for leadership in the next generation. A grandparent's love can provide a powerful experience of unconditional love for the grandchild, and in ways that help them believe in themselves and their talents. We can support their process, and show trust in their ability to figure things out in a spirit of right decision-making. We can also encourage children at an early age to share thoughts about the path they see for themselves. Sharing stories of how others resolved issues, came to decisions, or fulfilled dreams also provides opportunities for them to extrapolate threads of wisdom.

In addition to guiding children, we must remember that our personal lives are their laboratories as well. Like the learning we have gained from previous generations, we understand more and more the importance of future generations learning from our living. Our obligation to the magnificent emerging new generation is to embrace and live into our own healthy breadth. We will influence positive outcomes in an unfolding culture that will unequivocally rely on the wisdom and leadership of our grandchildren. Therefore, as women sage leaders, we must become the exemplary leaders, mentors, and models to show the way for the children of our planet.

Sages are watchful and seize opportunities to bring to

❦

light the potential they see in others. Jean Shinoda Bolen reframed Angeles Arrien's four guiding principles. Arrien succinctly advised us to show up, pay attention, speak our truth, and pray for the best outcome.[4] Bolen says that when our concern is for people we love, it is difficult to not be attached to the outcome. Sages may see that problems are likely to be encountered down a road our loved ones may take. So with that inner knowing in mind, with prayer for the best outcome, and with wisdom in our approach, we offer encouragement for the greatest potential to emerge. Interestingly, our own views of given situations may significantly change as we remain fully present, offering encouragement as needed, and being supportive of the emerging competencies of others. This becomes a reciprocal gift for us as continuously evolving visionaries.

Community. Women sages are interested in community participation. They become more interactive and collaborative after decades of livelihoods that may have created isolation. They find value in interacting with individuals, neighbors, and communities, discovering ways to talk, eat, play, and laugh together again. They may even seek new community tribes in which to belong and to establish deeper meaning in their lives.

Sages are influential in creating family within our communities. In earlier generations, the extended family was integral to the raising of children. Due to various factors, including the dynamics of mobility in our generation, family units are many times separated from family support. Laurie Bradley, a financial planner, says, "If women ruled the world, we'd bring back the extended family, or if family wasn't available, we'd set up our communities in a more integrated, extended family sort of way."[5] We can make new choices and identify creative ways to stay connected and support extended family, particularly in an era of superb communication opportunities. If our family is not intact, we can make choices to create communities in more integrated, extended family ways to proffer care and support in community.

Vocation. Many women in our current generation and generations to come, who are over the age of fifty, will continue working and defer retirement. This is due largely to longer life spans and economic and retirement plans that cannot support the years of living yet to unfold. However, with gifts of greater years and increasing quality in healthcare, aging allows us time to recreate work of the heart, so to speak, and envision avenues for continuing meaningful contributions for the good of society.

As our work continues, we will evolve beyond compulsive and unsatisfactory work habits and divisive competitive practices, and we will move into areas of genuinely inspired work and creativity. As women mature, they prefer to respond proactively to their inner knowing of personal passions. They focus on identifying contributions that are effective, supportive, and personally fulfilling. Such choices are reflected in what Rumi, thirteenth century Sufi poet, expressed as living from the inside out:

> When you do things from your soul,
> you feel a river moving in you, a joy.
> When actions come from another direction,
> the feeling disappears.[6]

Remembering this wisdom, sages will base vocational priorities on experiencing joy in work that nurtures their souls. Society will be faced, in turn, with the need to respond cooperatively and mutually with offerings through its institutions, organizations, and businesses.

Business. Women in the second half of life will develop businesses or work for businesses that flourish with a sense of heart-centered leadership. This requires people to lead from a true base of integrity to pursue visions with passion and compassion, and evoke the full potential of those with whom they come in contact. There is a focus from the principle of win-win-win. This means the employer, employee, and those served all benefit in the best possible way. They live from a spiritual base and are in business for their heart and soul as well as for financial success for themselves and for people with whom they work.

Industry. Savvy women who are sage leaders will be influential in conscientiously supporting the utilization or production of materials that are not harmful for the environment. They are proactive in responsible business practices that are implemented for sustainability and in harmony with nature. Progress will be made toward developing earth-friendly results. A life-affirming goal will be to find avenues that make food available for all people, because our values will shift from wasteful greed to meeting basic human needs. Nature is increasingly respected and protected, as we take greater care of the environment and its incredible resourcefulness.

Environment. Our culture has lost connections to spirit and nature caused by humanity's greater alignment to the material world and to technology. Nature is the source of our visions and centers us in truth. We, and our planet, are literally being destroyed because of materialism, not to mention wars and disease that result from such disharmony. The more nature is destroyed, the less able we are to live in balance and wisdom.

Elder Grandmother Agnes Baker Pilgrim says, "We have traded the welfare of future generations for immediate profit." In the teachings of *Grandmothers Counsel the World*, we are urged to examine our views of nature and respond affirmatively for her well-being. The Grandmothers believe that when we as a culture begin to understand the divinity in all things and the cosmological underpinnings of all life, that we will not take our beautiful Earth for granted any longer. They emphasize:

> Each one of us must decide now whether or not to live wisely and with a selfless love for the benefit of all. Will we choose to awaken to our higher consciousness in the face of dramatic Earth changes? Will we choose life?[7]

In addition, the accelerated extinction of species is what we have created with our own hands and under the current paradigm. There are various opportunities available to take action to protect nature and our environment. As we become more aware of problems on our planet such as global warming, destruction of rain forests, and lack of ecological sustainability, we will act consciously in our choices and commitments to make a difference. It is not to be taken lightly that we, as women, have profound collective power to live in harmony with nature.

Sustainability. Our lifestyles are positively altered when we live with an awareness of the influence our contributions have toward sustainability. When we respect Earth as a living organism, passion to protect her begins to emerge. As women sage leaders, we are prompted to weave new patterns of sustainability into the social fabric by first beginning with ourselves.

There are many possibilities to consider as we focus on changing our ways of living. We can begin practicing voluntary simplicity first by reducing our acquisitions and making thoughtful choices about what we need to own. Ecological sustainability is a broad area to explore so as to discover ways that we can make a difference to ensure our environment will remain viable for years to come. We can change the ways we live relative to environmental issues. Beginning may be as simple as investigating how to manage recyclable materials, or grow our own food, create compost, or limit excessive usage of products. Clearly, honoring and respecting nature as sacred is central to these issues.

Within the wellspring of wise knowledge of women sage leaders, we can successfully walk a path of sustainability. We can move through the scientific paradigm and mechanistic methodology, and access wisdom to show the way to living sustainably. Reaffirming the great interconnection of all relationships, we extend ourselves in this effort. The bottom line is that sage leaders are needed to create new and better ways of sustainable living in our society.

Healthcare. Supporting the acceptance of holistic healthcare can begin by expanding our choices for our own care. As we explore healthcare beyond traditional medicine, there are numerous alternatives to add to the options Western medicine offers. Women are leading this exploration using holistic practitioners who take into consideration the whole person. Their focus includes physical, mental, and spiritual aspects of care, when treating a health condition or promoting wellness.

Holistic professionals can be doctors, naturopaths, nurse practitioners, and chiropractors. Nutritionists, counselors, physical therapists, massage therapists, and energy practitioners can also be found in the category of holistic caregivers. These professionals employ complementary methods and alternative approaches to healthcare in their practices.

Beyond our own care, we may become influential in proposing ideas to others relative to our own successes. Furthermore, we can offer support for family members, friends, and neighbors in need, participating in their healthcare decisions to the extent they prefer to be supported. Of course, there are numerous ways to volunteer in compassionate service for care facilities, hospitals, daycare centers, and retirement residences.

Peaceful Inhabitancy. Women typically have an inborn capacity for inner peace and are able to open their hearts to reconciliation and healing. Louise Diamond believes that since women carry "the seeds of life to fruition," we are natural leaders for peace. She shares her views relative to her experiences with women around the world:

We nurture, we listen, we comfort, we maintain relationships. We are connected to our children—and to the life force. We intuitively understand when the circle of life is shattered and needs healing. Women get it. And because we get it, we are the mothers of peace—from the inside out.[8]

Even as "mothers of peace," because we are human, we encounter turbulent situations that can drain us of our energy and vitality. During those times, we can also find peace. Like the quiet in the eye of a hurricane, there is the capacity within us to reach a peaceful stillness deep in our hearts. It is a calm that mysteriously resides in our center.

Sages live as if "peace begins with me," because essentially it does. I once saw a plaque that succinctly stated this philosophy. It read, "Ultimately, we have just one moral duty: to reclaim large areas of peace in ourselves—more and more peace, and to reflect it toward others." With a peaceful presence, we gain a greater capacity to assist others in growing beyond difficulties emotionally and spiritually, and to celebrate their outcomes.

Inner peace can be a spiritual practice as well as a practical way of living. The Dalai Lama urges the daily spiritual practice of compassion, which he believes is a basis for world peace.[9] We must remember that as soon as children are born, they start learning from everything around them, including our teachings of peaceful presence. By this means, we are not only living examples, but are also planting seeds for a more peaceful inhabitancy on earth.

Justice. There are social conditions that absolutely warrant our attention. Women sages take action as they encounter opportunities to take a stand for justice. We express our intolerance of violence against women, children, and the elderly. We can support aspects of general feminism that positively influence the well-being of women. Once we open our hearts to matters for justice, doors will open that will catch our attention and call upon our wisdom.

Wise sages will encourage movement toward processes of justice integrated with processes for healing. Justice for all includes all people affected by injustice (such as individuals, neighborhoods, and communities), as well as those who practice unjust acts. How can we be effective in collaborating for fair outcomes? For example, justice that involves positive outcomes for diversity not only takes us closer to a more peaceful existence, but can also create a more beautiful tapestry of social experiences. Being proactive for justice is a courageous way to create a better society.

Politics. In order to emerge from warring political disarray on a national level, sage leaders will respond to guidance from visionaries providing counsel from a vantage point of peace. Can you imagine a governmental "Department of Defense" balanced with a "Department of Peace" providing wise perspectives for optimal peaceful and empowering results? In times of local, national, and global conflict, imagine peaceful and collaborative strategies for resolution instead of relying on sole practices of engaged aggression. Sages will continue to be proactive to employ a balance of men and women in political positions. And working collaboratively, their masculine and feminine voices will speak with wisdom to facilitate the business of our country.

Global Concerns. We must understand at a heart level that the soul of our nation and other world communities are as vital as the soul within every human being. As Carolyn Myss points out, an understanding of our human interconnectedness is as vital as our interconnectedness is with all of nature.[10] Our ethnicities, cultures, and communities are fabulously unique and diverse, and each is integral to the whole of our collective earthly existence. Women sages see that living in harmony with all living things—devoid of dominance—imparts a spirit of reverence. With such understanding, we embrace a cooperative spirit and live peacefully together, reaching higher levels of respect and acceptance with our worldwide brothers and sisters.

As we become more conscious of the impact that our own sage leadership has on others, we become more aware of the potential impact that other sage leaders have on our choices. Just as my mother, at the age of eighty-nine, learned how to use a computer and send letters via email to state senators, we too can be proactive at any age to express our concerns and opinions on government issues, locally and nationally. I am also impressed by the story of Doris Haddock, a political activist who gained national fame between the ages of eighty-eight and ninety. She walked across the country to gather support for a cause she believed in—campaigning for finance reform. Her goal was to arrive in Washington D.C. on her ninetieth birthday which she did on February 29, 2000.[11] We can continue to learn from the wise choices other women make relative to their commitments to create positive differences.

As sage leaders, we have great capacities to accomplish much if we keep our hearts open. When we free ourselves to be in relationship with what we love, and develop ways and structures to support that relationship, any place we go is the "promised land." To prosper in that *land*, it is critical that we learn to value ourselves with deeper respect and honor, and not allow negativity to take hold of us during challenging situations. As we keep devoted to our personal truth and stand firm on our spiritual principles, we will continue to gain greater trust in our inner knowing. Furthermore, we will flourish with deeper understanding as we work with, and are in harmony with, the sacred knowledge that exists on Earth. Thereby, we plant the seeds to birth our new living legacy.

Manifesting Fulfillment

As women walk into the aging arena, our search for meaning in life shifts. We are finite, and we do not have unlimited time to do what we want with our lives. We have the potential to take action, or not to act, remembering inaction is a decision in and of itself. Since we can choose our actions, we can also influence our own destiny. Wisdom teaches us that as we increase awareness of choices available in our later decades, we also increase our sense of responsibility for the consequences of our choices.

As we make choices focusing our intention on manifesting greater fulfillment, hopefully we realize the incredible value of learning from other women. They are truly precious resources for trans-generational relationships. As we learn that we are always subject to meaninglessness, loneliness, emptiness, guilt, and isolation, we also have choices relative to these conditions of the human experience. Much of the time these experiences become more challenging as we get older. Yet we still have opportunities to choose how we relate to others.

This point is poignantly depicted in my last visit with my beloved Aunt Peggy before her death transition. She was a vital woman throughout her life, and the woman that I looked to with aspiration. Peggy was, and remains, my mentor, my teacher, and my heroine. She lived a simple life, and shared her gifts quietly. She could have been an influential ambassador, a famous and renowned artist, scientist, composer, musician, farmer, politician, physician, minister, and more, if her stage had been broader. Yet in the middle of rural Nebraska, she was all of the above in her quiet, courageous, and confident manner. She was like an unknown Hildegard von Bingen. As I was growing up, she was the smartest woman I knew. Surprisingly to me, she became diminished by dementia in her nineties. Yet even in what is deemed a negative human condition, I witnessed that she—at the age of ninety-six—still attempted to relate to others.

Understanding that my aunt's condition was fragile, I traveled to the Midwest to see her. A nurse directed me to a sunroom in the Alzheimer's wing where she then lived. As I approached the sunroom, I saw a circle of wheelchairs where such seasoned souls gathered. My eyes searched for her, and then I saw her crumpled body supported by two physical therapists. She swayed like a rag doll, suspended by a strap around her belly. Barely shuffling one foot and then the other, she struggled to keep her chin up off her chest. Another resident called from across the room, "Stop! You'll hurt her! She doesn't want to walk!" The lady remained openly agitated, spewing empathic commands in spite of a therapist's attempt to reassure her. My aunt was finally released from seemingly futile physical therapy efforts. One of the physical therapists assisted her back to a wheelchair. She was clearly exhausted.

A nurse spoke to her, "Do you want to go over and visit with Marilyn? Marilyn is here."

"Marilyn?" she uttered, looking up and questioning. My heart ached for this very influential woman in my life. I loved her dearly, and the rawness of the moment erupted into a volcano of contained emotions. In recent years, she slipped away from the reality in which she once lived independently. It was torment for me to see her decline to such a difficult existence, seemingly stimulated mostly by drawing circles on her thigh with her right third finger.

The nurse pushed her chair toward me across the room, away from the circle of wheelchairs. I greeted her and felt privileged to have one more opportunity to hug her and say, "I love you." She briefly engaged and then her eyes turned downward; she then appeared to retreat. I could not guess what she was thinking. I waited, and then said, "It looks like you're thinking about something."

"Yes," she said. I waited with her in her silence. Her fingers worked around a button and buttonhole at the bottom of her colorful blouse, and then she appeared to escape into slumber. With my hand on her knee, I waited as time passed.

I remembered when I was twelve and my uncle died suddenly from a heart attack while working in the fields. His sudden death was a shock to my aunt and our family. It seemed like only a few years ago that she sat in a stupor of grief in my father's rocking chair that afternoon. Yet she gathered herself together and soon thereafter embarked on a world trip. Her horizons broadened as she courageously created a new chapter in her life that would not have been thought possible. When she returned home, she had a multitude of speaking engagements to teach about the living and political conditions she found during her travels. Her experiences were the first encounters many people in her audiences had beyond their own communities.

Suddenly, I returned to the present moment as I heard a woman singing and her harsh voice echoing loudly throughout the room. Another resident clasped her hands over her ears clearly annoyed by the singing. Demands were shouted from the longing mouths of others in the circle, while others simply sat silently. I watched a man who came to visit his wife reach awkwardly across her twisted body crumpled in a lounger and tenderly caress her parted lips. With her eyes gazing toward the ceiling, I noticed a slight upturn appear at the corners of her mouth, seemingly appreciating the presence of her sweetheart.

I extended my hand and held Aunt Peggy's soft chin in my palm, and leaned close to kiss her forehead. My heart was so full of love for her. I whispered, "I'll love you forever."

She opened her eyes and, looking up, slightly smiled and replied, "And the same for you, Dear." It was as if that was her benediction for me to carry in my heart for the rest of my life. We sat for some time together, quietly, holding each other's hand. She seemed comfortable and content.

In those moments, I resolved in my heart that I had completed what I needed to say to this wonderful, lovely woman. I released her hand and pushed her wheelchair back into the circle of other precious ones. The sound of a deep and sudden burst of my own emotional breath filled my ears. Although I was uncertain what she had left to do or say in this world, I recognized that the courage and will to live is mysterious and cannot be reasoned. Gazing around the circle of wheelchairs, I realized that the power of love penetrates deep and does *not* require cognition. Its powerful energy flows naturally and is a gift to be exchanged regardless of the circumstances in which it prevails. Did I manifest fulfillment during the time I spent with my aunt? That was not my intention; however, unexpectedly even in those difficult circumstances, it was the result.

Sage wisdom speaks to us when we slow down and discover meaning even in suffering. Even in human suffering, the negative aspects of life can be turned into human achievements by the stand and attitude that women take in the face of any situation. Sage wisdom underscores the prevalence of love regardless of the human condition. It speaks to the bravery women demonstrate in facing pain, guilt, despair, or death. With intuition and wisdom, the sage challenges her situation and thus triumphs with new strength, insight, and awareness.

To expand our awareness is to increase our capacity to live fully and manifest fulfillment. Viktor Frankl, an existential theorist, proposed that as human beings we could reflect and make choices because we are capable of self-awareness. Greater self-awareness is impetus for greater possibilities for fulfillment. Yet finding meaning or manifesting fulfillment is not something that we can directly search for and obtain through self-awareness alone. Similar to pleasure, meaning must be pursued obliquely, so to speak. Frankl believed that finding meaning in life is a by-product of "engagement," which is a commitment to creating, loving, working, and building.[12] Therefore, when women continue to create from their center of wisdom, love unconditionally, engage in the work of their hearts, and build new vistas, a sense of fulfillment emerges. Meaning and fulfillment are not automatically bestowed on us, but are results of our searching, discovering, and ultimate offerings.

Additionally, if in our later decades we have few regrets and feel personally worthwhile, then we have manifested fulfillment. Failure to achieve a sense that our lives have been valuable and meaningful can lead to feelings of despair, hopelessness, guilt, resentment, and self-rejection. The ultimate later-life stage in human development according to Erikson's Psychosocial Stages is the challenge of integrity versus despair.[13] This is a time of adjusting to the discrepancy between one's dreams and one's actual accomplishments. The challenge of this later-life stage calls us to take the initiative to live in the second half of life from the depths of our womanly wisdom. It asks us to walk in our unique personal authenticity regardless of any discrepancies between prior dreams and accomplishments.

It is essential to remember that each woman has unique wisdom that only the days of her own living could have manifested. It is a wisdom that the collective consciousness needs. Therefore, it is your choice and magnificent opportunity to reach down in the heart of your soul, grasp hold of wisdom, and never let go, as reflected in the magnificent poetry of Makeda, Queen of Sheba, written in ca. 1000 B.C.E.

> I fell
> because of wisdom,
> but was not destroyed:
> through her I dived
> into the great sea,
> and in those depths
> I seized
> a wealth-bestowing pearl.
>
> I descended
> like the great iron anchor
> used to steady ships
> in the night on rough seas,
> and holding up the bright lamp
> that I there received,
> I climbed the rope
> to the boat of understanding.

While in the dark sea,
I slept,
and not overwhelmed there,
dreamt: a star
blazed in my womb.

I marveled
at that light,
and grasped it,
and brought it up to the sun.
I laid hold upon it,
and will not let it go.[14]

As we search for meaning and fulfillment, it is imperative we open to the wisdom and ongoing potential of our visions. A profound example that comes to mind is the vision of Susan B. Komen's sister, Nancy Brinker. After Susan's death from breast cancer, Nancy made a commitment to make a difference for women relative to research, causes, treatment, and the search for the cure for breast cancer. Now, with worldwide participation, the organization is the most progressive grassroots network for breast cancer survivors and activists (komen.org).

Since its inception, the Komen organization has sustained a strong commitment to supporting research that will identify and deliver cures for breast cancer. This commitment has resulted in important progress that has contributed to every major advance in breast cancer research over the past thirty-five years. With increasing investments over time, Komen is now the largest non-government funder of breast cancer research. The commitment to energize science to find the cures started their very first year (1982) with just one grant for $28,000. By the beginning of the second decade, they were funding more than twenty research grants annually and just seven years later were funding more than one hundred research grants annually. To date, the organization has invested more than $2.5 billion in groundbreaking research, community health outreach, advocacy, and programs in more than thirty countries.

Another remarkable vision manifested Seeds of Compassion (seedsofcompassion.org) This movement came about after a meeting between Dan Kranzler, founder of the Kirlin Charitable Foundation and the Venerable Lama Tenzin Dhonden in 2005, and resulted in the Seeds of Compassion Conference in Seattle in April 2008. The event marked the beginning of a collaboration that would increase public awareness and would empower a call to action, focusing on both local and global needs for the social and emotional well-being of our children. It was viewed as a grassroots initiation for an emerging global Compassion Movement that would provide tools and programs that nurture and empower children, families, and communities to be compassionate members of society.

Many programs have sprouted out of the Seeds of Compassion event. For example, Compassionate Action Network evolved as a "sprout of compassion." CAN aims to focus attention on what we do in the world, in all of our institutions—schools, foundations, community organizations, nonprofits, small businesses and corporations, hospitals, unions, and professional associations. This action network also encourages integration of compassion in our families, neighborhoods, prisons and halfway houses, faith and spiritual communities, government (city councils, state legislatures and legislators, Congress and national lawmakers), and the military—to adopt and promote compassion as the guiding principle.

Seattle made history by being the first city to affirm the Charter for Compassion, and making a commitment to a ten-year Campaign for Compassionate Cities. Charter of Compassion is committed to building a worldwide network of Compassionate Communities. It envisions a richly diverse "network of networks," people from every sector—business, healthcare, education, government, faith and interfaith, peace and non-violence, science and research, social services, the arts, and those working to preserve the environment. It welcomes those who will bring compassion to everything they do. They embrace those who will take responsibility for igniting the compassion of the general community to care for each other and for the well-being of all members of the community. Members include all ages from birth through childhood, adolescence and adulthood, to old age and death.

In an interview with Marilyn Turkovich, director for a Compassionate Community in Puget Sound, she stated that as of 2015, The Charter for Compassion International works with over 300 cities in 50 countries. They assist in creating multiple year plans addressing issues in their communities. While the Charter does not prescribe any one path, Ms. Turkovich says, "It does recommend that the process be designed and carried out by a diverse and inclusive coalition of people so that all voices within the community are heard, and significant issues are addressed."

You cannot predict the power of your own visions, nor the influence you could have in creating good in the world.

As you envision living your legacy as a sage leader, begin to trust the fertile ground of your visions. Have faith that manifesting fulfillment comes from your willingness to take another next step. You will never be able to predict the ripple effect of actions that you take. Just believe that the world is waiting to welcome your gifts. Sharing those gifts becomes your living legacy.

Imparting a Mentoring Spirit

In the second half of life, there is a need to go beyond self and family and to help the next generation. Failure to achieve a sense of generativity can lead to psychological and spiritual inertia. The main task of generativity is to guide the next generation through our acts of care. As sages consider the abundance of ways to give to others, one of the most profound gifts we can offer is a mentoring spirit.

We can look to traditional societies where the grandmothers are the ones who are looked up to as guardians to watch over the physical and spiritual survival of the family, and thus the tribe. They are the keepers of the teachings and rituals that allow their tribe to flourish. They uphold the social order. In many tribes around the world, grandmothers are consulted before major decisions in the tribe are made, decisions that even include whether or not to go to war. They are intergenerational mentors who are held in high esteem.

In Western society, mentoring companionships are not prevalent or part of a relational paradigm. However, making a commitment to be a mentor, or trusted guide, is a valuable offering. A sage mentor tells the truth about her life and is a woman who has walked the path we or others want to take. As mentor companions, they use their familiarity with the landscape of time to reassure others when they become afraid or lose heart. They are open to sharing that they have also been through similar circumstances that the other person is experiencing. With a broader vantage point, mentors are able to see potential in others that they may not be able to see in themselves.

One of the greatest gifts of grace and love as a mentor is the experience as a grandparent. The relationship between grandparent and grandchild can be positively effectual in supporting a child's growth of self-confidence and self-discovery. There will no doubt also be various occasions for us to share our positions, ideas, and opinions that may be helpful based on wisdom gained from our years of experience. We can use our familiarity with various life, social, and relational skills as we companion with our grandchildren. We can also be effective through our meditations and prayers, holding them in a spirit of highest good. Certainly, we can send positive thoughts into any situation. Of course, for the grandparent, the child fosters experiences once again for awe, wonder, play, laughter, and adventure.

While grandparenting provides significant interconnectedness between generations, there are other meaningful ways to connect with younger people. We must understand that it is not necessary to have biological grandchildren in order to be significant, influential mentors for children. We can serve as long as we live in some capacity as mentors regardless of whether we are grandmothers or not. As we keep watchful hearts for

children's best welfare, we can also hold high our belief in
their greatness. I convey this philosophy in the poem "For
the Children":

> May you always have passion for life
> and revere all living things.
> May you always be inspired
> to bring your unique creative energies into form.
> May you also honor your power of choice
> and respect the greatness
> that resides within you.
>
> May you always be tempted to courageously glimpse
> into new depths of your soul,
> embrace the magnificence of your bright light,
> and not be afraid of your own dark corners,
> remembering wisdom of the half moon
> teaches the necessity of dark and light,
> which is inherent to wholeness.
>
> May you tenderly care for your body,
> trust your mind, listen intently to your spirit.
> May you understand that you
> are the author of your wisdom, your joy and love.
> May you live with a peaceful heart
> and a healthy discontent to continuously seek,
> ever-transcending into your best version of you.
>
> I pray that you intuit that the world needs you,
> your contributions,
> your choices,
> and your legacy.

I pray that you are confident
that your life matters
and shines forth with inspired purpose.

I pray that whatever or whomever your god is,
or becomes,
there is an unshakable knowing deep in your soul
of a loving Divine Presence in the universe—
or multiverses, for all we know,
that also resides eternally at the core of your being,
caring deeply about you and the flow of your life.

Last, and not least, remember . . .
I will always be with you
as you progressively learn to live in freedom
as your *true Self*.
You will never be alone.
I will always be in tandem, by your side,
in this world and in the next.[15]

Our contributions as loving mentors are essential and limited only by our lack of vision. I remember the vision of one elderly woman to make a difference for babies in intensive care at a children's hospital where I was an intern many years ago. She proposed her idea of creating a "Grandmothering Program." The hospital directors accepted her proposal and took action to create guidelines to move forward with her vision. They collaborated to create a means for older women to visit the neonatal intensive care unit on a daily basis to touch, hold, and rock selected infants. The "grandmother volunteers" were also available to older children, further extending their gifts by companioning, reading, and storytelling. For many children, the Grandmothering Program provided their first initial opportunities for deep, consistent, harmonious human nurturing. They often established a trusting relationship before their families could.

Women sage mentors give a lot of importance to developing and maintaining relationships in general. An eighty-four-year-old friend of mine, Louise, spent much of her time with younger women. She was quick to offer her rationale. Louise found that younger female friends inspired her with fresh ideas, engaged in stimulating conversations, and complained less than most women her age. She further shared that while younger friends helped her frequently, she also had many opportunities to reciprocate with her unique ability to help others discover and believe in the value of their own unique abilities. This was her life work in theatre. She was the founder of the Bainbridge Island Performing Arts Center. Although Louise was never an actress, she said her gift was to find people who did not yet know their acting potential, or had not yet claimed their artistic abilities. She had a keenness for identifying talent from costuming and stage setting to acting. Louise believed her purpose was to be a "finder" of talent for community enjoyment and pleasure through the arts. Louise lived with a mentoring spirit every day.

Focusing on mentoring relationships also includes caring intensely about spiritual and psychological development of those whose lives we touch. Sages personally continue to be open to their own nurturance, as well as honoring the importance of spirituality or religion in the lives of others. We seize opportunities to nurture children, grandchildren, families, and friends with an inner knowing that our collective spiritual and psychological health impacts the well-being of our society.

There is a deep sense of satisfaction and fulfillment when we give of ourselves and share our personal resources. *Spirituality and Health* reported that being highly generative is a sign of psychological health and maturity.[16] Individuals have higher levels of happiness and well-being, and have lower levels of depression and anxiety. While mentoring companionships are good for our personal and global families, they are also good for us individually.

Honoring Intergenerational Connectedness

An evolving developmental theory for older women defines the self in relation to an interdependent society. The older woman striving for expansion of the self in relationships with others experiences a more developed self within more multifaceted connections.[17] This idea does not focus on the Western developmental theory of separation and independence as the goal of human growth. Understanding this concept deepens our knowing of interconnectedness. We are perpetually in relation to something else that in turn is related to something else, and so on to the furthest reaches of the Universe.

At some point in the second half of life comes the realization of how profoundly we are connected to a stream of previous and future generations. From inherited legacies, myths, and legends, and from anthropologists and historians, we learn that the elders of society are the teachers of tradition. With these roles, they are the teachers of new ways, the keepers of ancestral values, and providers of continuity. This contributes to the interdependence of all age groups.

All generations crave knowledge of their past. We need long-lived narratives and stories of human relationships with historical depth. Myths, folk tales, proverbs, stories, celebrations, and songs tell us who we are and who we can be. Documenting our lives and history is a vital gift to successive generations. We want to know about the land and people that first nurtured us, where our ancestors came from, and about the experiences that shaped them and, ultimately, us.

As women sages, we must not "leave" until we tell our stories. For in the telling, we not only hear our stories, but also hear those stories of our mothers and grandmothers. We must not leave until we free ourselves from misinterpretations, as our stories reach back in time before we were constrained by myths.[18] In freeing the myths, we will also claim our freedom and liberation as women sages. Furthermore, we must not leave this life without acknowledging our glory, and freeing our voices to shout out the truth and courage of our lifetime.

Our longer life span now offers opportunities never before available for conversation, healing, and intimacy between generations. Attempting to create understanding between generations is itself an act of love, even if we do not know what will be the outcome. We give the gifts we want to give and address the issues that cause separation. We attempt to make peace with one another, beginning with the process of making peace with ourselves. We may be willing to pay the price of taking a bold stand to heal generational tragedy as evidenced by physical, sexual, emotional, and verbal abuse. We may face off with alcoholism, or attempt to slay the dragons of mental illness, knowing well the interconnectedness of generations. When we are able to mourn our pain and regrets, and come to peace with ourselves, we contribute to the legacy of putting an end to negative impacts on the next generation. We can truly engage in various occasions of celebration and honor our generational interconnectedness.

Our new story is being birthed. Our greatest challenges are to preserve and sustain life on the planet and to find new ways for spiritual and psychological breadth, as well as harmonious coexistence. The world needs us right now to birth and live our Fire of Vision. Sages realize the urgency of this work.

Indeed, this is the time to attend to the wisdom of our visions and to take action to manifest images that arise from the heart of the sage. I am reminded of a vision that came to me during a poetry guided meditation a few years ago. Reflections of fond childhood moments came to my mind. Images of my beloved brother who died in early adulthood prompted me to capture memories through poetic expression. It became apparent to me that layers of wisdom are revealed throughout time. I sensed elements of wisdom coming from a deep place. The images precipitated questions about my potential gifts to others in this sacred time:

In Our Sacred Time

My brother died young
at thirty-five.

❤

He used to ask me,
again and again,
for another glass of water.
I pretended to not want to—
yet, I adored him and
simply fetched more water.

As kids, at mealtimes
we lingered after others
left the worn kitchen table.
Our child eyes danced
in the space between us
and we would simply laugh.

It was our sacred time—
glasses full of water,
hands banging the table,
air echoing our laughter,
fire in our child hearts,
joy from our kindred souls.

I used to ask my brother,
again and again,
for advice about life.
I trusted him—yet knew
somehow wisdom came
from my own deep well.

Now, staring through
the windowpane beyond
the old kitchen table
in the abandoned room

in my mind, once again
memories usher grief.

My tender heart quickens . . .
How might I bring
life-giving gifts to others
in this dear, sacred time?
I listen—seeing in my mind
his kind, benevolent heart.

Love and respect others—
bring water for their glasses,
strong metal for their tables,
sustain pure air for laughter,
tend fire for their passion,
share joy for hurting hearts.

His sweetness welled inside
as I breathed my prayer,
Lead me to those who need
life-sustaining gifts
like water . . . like joy
like we had in our sacred time.

And my brother
simply whispered, *Yes,*
as I felt him next to me
sitting in the empty chair,
gazing out the window
in my mind.[19]

It is indeed our sacred time. As women sage leaders, we need to ask the questions: "Will what I give be good for the seventh generation into the future?" "Will what I give be good for the planet?" We must connect with our inner wisdom and the knowledge gained from years of living, and stay true to our understanding. We do not stand alone in this courageous work; every woman is needed to weave new patterns in the social fabric of aging. The wisdom we have to create new ground for women's aging issues is the guiding story for the future.

Our Fire of Vision involves envisioning a better world, fulfilling our generative goals, imparting a mentoring spirit, and supporting a sustainable future. Considering these views, we are sensitized to the sacredness of life. Truthfully, I believe the future looks to each of us for hope. For the benefit of our culture's maturity, it is necessary to recognize we are called forth by the archetype of an emerging *wise spirit*, the path of wisdom-in-action and the ways of living our Sagessence. We can begin to celebrate our living legacies as inspired by Mary Radmacher-Hershey's poem:

Living Eulogy

She danced.
She sang.
She took.
She gave.
She served.
She loved.
She created.
She dissented.

She enlivened.
She saw.
She grew.
She sweated.
She changed.
She learned.
She laughed.
She shed her skin.
She bled on the pages of her days.
She walked through walls.
She lived with intention.[20]

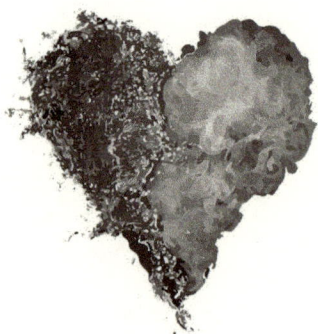

Chapter 6

Tending Fire in the Heart

♥

Tending Fire in the Heart
fosters sage wisdom by honoring our life story,
by exalting our female wisdom,
by revering our Sagessence,
and by living sagacity-in-action.

As a woman awakens fire in her heart, she ignites her Sagessence. It is her wise spirit that is the ultimate beauty of her feminine fullness. It reflects her illumination as a sage leader living from the center of her unique wisdom, a rich wisdom gained from living her sacred journey. Sagessence can also be described as *wise spirit in action*. As a sage, this kind of action becomes our individual work. Yet as Sagessence emerges in women awakening across our country and around the world, we find community and support in ongoing opportunities as we connect and celebrate with other women.

As we come together physically, mentally, and spiritually around a fire that ignites a sage movement, let us remember the power of women gathering with women. It is through supporting each other's unique stories, honoring our rich life wisdom, and sharing our own liberating images of aging that we will strengthen in our efforts. There is strength in women collectively supporting women's stories. Such support is not only an act of honoring and validating each other. It also precipitates rich possibilities of ongoing re-envisioning and proactive choices to manifest meaningful fulfillment and contributions in the second half of life. Exponentially, it can also precipitate contentment in our hearts, as well as stimulate positive change in cultural views of aging.

Honoring Our Stories

Sages are not just women who have reached their fifties and beyond. They are women who are doing so in a conscious and intentional way. As sages, we look back over our lives to see the paths we have traveled, and then look forward to see how we can contribute to the world. I relate Marian Van Eyk McCain's following comments to our feminine journey as well as to the woman sage, "She has not only lived long enough to acquire both knowledge and wisdom, but she knows and values the difference between them and she is prepared to go on acquiring the one and distilling the other."[1]

Powerful wisdom and self-liberation come when we take time to review our life with all its joy and awe, sorrow and lament. This is not always easily accomplished. As we revisit the events of our life, reinterpretation may result in our experiencing elements of satisfaction, joy, failure, and/or heartfelt misgivings. Fulfillment is sensed when we can view our lives with a sense of personal truth, love, compassion, and vision. In so doing, we can experience each unfolding moment as sacred time. We sense Divine significance throughout our days, and gain confidence in our continued life as we intentionally make decisions from the center of our wisdom.

It is helpful to approach our respective life reviews by owning the accumulating wisdom we have gained throughout our decades. In *A Woman's Book of Life*, Joan Borysenko discusses feminine life cycles common to all women. Her work beautifully depicts the evolving wisdom inherent in a woman's life. Examining our life stages is certainly beneficial to attain deeper insights, keeping in mind that our lives are an ever-evolving spiral whereby we may repeatedly come to epochs that are similar to prior experiences throughout our lives. However, we never experience those times again in quite the same way. This is particularly true when we acknowledge the natural wisdom we are born with, and integrate ongoing wisdom that emerges from our life course. To gain further appreciation and knowledge, it is indeed helpful to review generally our typical progression of womanly wisdom.

We were born with a *natural wisdom*.[2] During our first life decade as children, we no doubt demonstrated a clear appreciation of the present moment, which was truly instinctual. Many of us perceived things that adults did not perceive, like angels and imaginary friends. It was typical to think intuitively and holistically, and to live in somewhat of a dream state with expanded views of reality.

Typically, by the end of our early childhood, we had developed gifts of empathy that we naturally imparted in our relationships with other people, other beings, and different environments. As young children, we gained interdependent perception and awareness. Generally, this sensitivity offered potential to continue throughout our development, expanding both through experience and continuing biological changes for the remainder of our life cycle. When we, as young girls, were recognized and encouraged for the remarkable strengths we had, our strengths naturally unfolded in our personal and collective lives.

The second decade encompassed our adolescence and initial transformation as young women. This was the decade when we attempted to resolve a conflict between the power *to be* and the power *to please*. We were immersed in the relational world preparing for a role in sustaining interdependent connectedness between ourselves and others, and between people and nature. During teenage years, we became conscious of body image, searched for identity, and either found or lost our voice.

This decade was also when we typically began menstrual periods and moved through the first amazing female metamorphosis. We experienced and expressed emotions cyclically. We learned that our society usually frowned upon our negative emotions, and judgment prevailed relative to the challenging aspects of female emotions. However, relative to the menstrual interval, we were typically able to release difficult emotions that may have been building up all month. Borysenko says, "This emotional housecleaning is wrongly viewed as bitchiness or complaining, but when seen rightly and heeded, it may be a valuable stress reducer and guide to what we need to change or pay attention to so that our lives will run more smoothly."[3]

Many women experience enhanced intuitive capacity, perceptions, and potential creativity during premenstrual and menstrual cycles. These elements can be viewed as contributors to an emerging depth of wisdom in this decade. Indeed, during this time, our first feminine transition began to emerge as we prepared for young adulthood.

For women who are fifty years and older today, the third decade—our twenties—was the time we typically left home, manifested committed relationships, mated, birthed children, and became mothers. A tricky potential dilemma was that the development of a strong sense of self-in-relation occurred for us in adolescence and, in the best-case scenarios, began to mature only in our twenties. While not yet mastered, this limitation may have created difficulties for many of us in choosing an emotionally healthy partner or, on the other hand, being an emotionally healthy partner ourselves. We may have given our power over to another, or erroneously believed that we could change our significant other into someone more suitable for us.

The quality of relationships that we developed during this decade was supported by what we, as young women, had already learned, and with warnings about what things we had not yet mastered. Typically, we looked to happiness, creativity, compassion, and a satisfying sense of mutual growth in relationships. When these elements were not present in our relationships as young women, emotional feedback may have prompted a change in course of our thoughts and behaviors.

The gift of the thirties transition was the process of values clarification and, according to Borysenko, is the first of many that occur throughout the feminine life cycle.[4] As young women, we wrestled with what was important in our lives and what success looked like. We may have wondered what we could provide for our children, family, and the world. It may have become important to identify our personal spiritual beliefs. This was a time to attend to old baggage, to clear our way, and attend to creative opportunities for the future.

The thirties was also a time when we, as young women, struggled to resolve the adolescent dilemma of reclaiming the ability to speak for oneself, if indeed our voice was previously silenced. This era was a time to do what we needed to do without feeling as if we were being selfish. We learned the wisdom of compromise, balance, and reevaluating the foundation of our life structure. We deepened our ability to connect with others, to nurture, and to make decisions based on the present and future, instead of on the past. This actually may have precipitated through our spirit of mothering.

As women enter their forties, they come into an era when wisdom of authentic self-authority clearly evolves. Our second transformation is at midlife during which time we reflect on our early adult life, examine what is most meaningful and important, and then plan our life structure for the second half of life.[5] During this decade, our womanly wisdom leads us to resolve what may have kept us from enjoying the life structures we carefully put into place. This is a decade to make new priorities. We may complete prior developmental phases that may not yet be fully mastered and that involve working on emotional healing. The need for healing often becomes evident when recurring problems in relationships signal that something within us needs to be resolved. This is the work of transforming old wounds into wisdom, from something considered old and worthless into something precious and enduring.

If we have balanced our priorities and healed old emotional scars by the end of early adulthood, we are in an excellent position to go through the metamorphosis of midlife and continue on into deeper authenticity, relationality, power, and service that are all fundamental to the last half of life. Major life changes may take place during this time such as relationship structures, divorce, careers, and children emptying our nest. There comes a realization that no experiences from which we gained gifts of understanding and compassion, even difficult ones, have been worthless. Whether we consciously realize it or not, we grieve on various levels those losses experienced in our young adulthood. We have reached various levels of healing in areas of our lives. We may exude a sense of peace and openheartedness and become less prone to judge others, situations, and circumstances. We have learned to balance many different life tasks. Our bodies move toward another female metamorphosis of ending fertility and changes precipitated by menopause.

Deeper questions come to consciousness as we attempt to clarify who we are, what we treasure, what is the meaning and purpose of our life, and to identify true happiness. Our authenticity arises from our process of self-examination and self-reflection. The mid-life crisis appears to arise from a transition created when we evaluate what has been in the past and what lies ahead. Our lives are changed dramatically in the wake of such an examination. We establish the new foundation for remarkable wisdom that is about to emerge in the next cycle of life. We begin to develop our male side, or animus—our *feminine brawn*.[6] And we start to sense the deeper, intuitive, creative wisdom that has always been within us.

Our significant metamorphosis and emerging wisdom is birthed out of menopause. There are intense changes in hormone levels that typically precipitate concurrent symptoms of hot flashes, interrupted sleep, fatigue, and night sweats. Joan Borysenko describes hot flashes as "the power source for the iron foundry in which an expanded feminine power is being forged."[7] Menopause may be considered an initiation into what can be the most powerful, exciting, and fulfilling era of a woman's life. As adolescents, we gained the physiological capacity to nurture children. Now, we gain the capacity to mother the larger world beyond typical boundaries of family.

As women approach their fifties, they come to the portal of the second half of life. Hilariously, our society has viewed women transitioning into the second half of life as a negative time of change because this is the end of productive years. However, in truth this is a time that allows women to become more sensuous and creative than ever before in their lives. We dream more vividly; we gain increased sureness in judgment, stronger intuition, self-confidence, self-integrity, and self-compassion. We demonstrate a kind of fierce, cut-through-it-all wisdom that helps us break old patterns and fuels us toward deeper authenticity. When a woman is emotionally mature and psychologically healthy, a new boldness emerges that is channeled into personal, family, and social causes. This manner of boldness fosters values of relationality and interdependence.

By this time in a woman's life, we have come to an appreciation of what Borysenko names the "feminine triad of love."[8] This triad involves: a) the expression of self-in-relation through which two people help bring one another into expanded states of creativity and happiness; b) the awareness of peacefulness that comes from authenticity; and c) service that involves concerns for the environment, the preservation of the planet for future generations with gifts of altruism that make a real difference. As we embrace these emerging values of love, serenity, and service, we concurrently expand our own happiness and quality of life.

Many women in their sixties integrate their passion into action through service and altruism. They identify who it is that they most are drawn to serve in utilizing their personal wisdom and resources. With a sense of interdependence, they gain understanding that what we do for anyone else, we also do for ourselves. Without service to others, we would not have the opportunity to become better human beings. By putting our wise spirits into action, every act of kindness and compassion toward others gets multiplied when we, in turn, pass it on. One by one, we make the world a better place. By remaining active and involved in the world and by using our voices, we can truly become sages in action.

The perspective of aging as a progressive loss of function is generally true only for people who stop functioning. We have all heard the phrase, "use it or lose it," which is a powerful truth for later decades of life. There is relatively little biology to consider because, at least with current scientific research, physical development is essentially complete, although the brain continues to create new pathways in response to intellectual stimulation until the very moment of our death. The ideal is to preserve the biological function that we have matured into at menopause and to continue our psychological, interpersonal, and spiritual development.

Between the ages of sixty and sixty-five, another period

of retrospection of our life and planning for our elder years occurs. This involves another life review, so to speak, and taking account of what changes we want to initiate for more fulfilling lives. It is a time when wise women become exemplary in their ability to convey truth with the relational skills needed in order for their message to be heard. In fact, sages of our time may be the foremothers of an emerging time in which the art of relationality rebuilds balance in a burdened world.

The seventies typically bring experiences of greater losses and changing life experiences.[9] Such circumstances can result from careers that have ended, retirement life, moving from homes to retirement communities or apartments, and inevitable deaths of family members and friends. We typically cope with the same coping strategies we learned from our earlier life. Many times, this is with resiliency, and other times women may need to establish new coping skills. Hopefully, we rely on our strong social support and optimistic attitudes. We continue to be responsible for what we need, with particular attention to nurturing mental and physical stimulation. Our society typically views this time as the era of the inevitable miseries of aging, rather than as opportunities to see what we are made of and to provide a model for our families, friends, and the culture at large. As we experience perpetual endings, we can also anticipate perpetual beginnings. Our endings, such as the death of a spouse, can result in an entirely new and exciting life opening.

Perhaps the greatest gift of these wisdom years is a renewed understanding of how important a network of close friends is to our health, happiness, and longevity. A great percentage of women in the eighth decade are still healthy and can continue to grow psychologically, intellectually, spiritually, and relationally. An active and vital life still remains.

We can either focus on negative aspects of our aging that are culturally familiar, or we can concentrate on how we can create a more positive life. Although there are elements of later life that are indeed concerning, I consider differing attitudes in the following poem:

Aging

What is this journey of aging—
this unfamiliar dwelling place?

Is it like a house of loneliness
with quiet, cluttered rooms
where pictures on the walls
reflect loss of family, friends
And the tattered ledger
in the marred old oak desk
still guards notes in margins
There, where doodled dreams
still remain formless because
there simply is not enough
money in lint-edged pockets
for basic needs, let alone
for pipedreams anymore?

Or,

Is it an extraordinary voyage…
a ship setting sail on new seas

with a key banging in the berth
There, to open a treasure chest
its bejeweled latch opening to
the sage—maturity, wisdom
more time, more freedom, and
satisfying forgotten dreams?
I don't really know as yet,
I've not been this old before
But, I choose to climb aboard
with a keen ear to listening
for the knocking of that key.[10]

As we become more acutely aware of lessening time, and our own inevitable death, a gift to ourselves is possible by taking an opportunity to come to terms with the way we are living. Are there things we want to accomplish? What are the important things we can still do for ourselves and for others? Are we stagnating? A reality check at this age prompts these questions and can lead to choices that can help us to create lives that are more satisfying.

As women entering our eighties, we have completed a series of general transitions in life during which we reexamined what has gone before. The first transition was at the end of adolescence as we prepared for entry into early adulthood. The second transition was at midlife during which we reflected on our early adult life, examined what was most meaningful and important, and then planned our life structure for our second half of life. Between sixty and sixty-five, there came another period of retrospection and planning for the rest of our years. A fourth period of retrospection occurs in our eighties. However, rather than planning the next phase of our life, we begin to extract the meaning of our lifetime as a whole, typically with profound spiritual integration. Each previous transition revolved around a core question of identifying what we had learned and how it would serve us in the next phase of life.

In many conversations I have had with women between the years of eighty and ninety, it became clear there was a realization that the next phase of their life was indeed death. Reflecting on life as an integrative whole had become paramount. Several heartfelt questions may be asked during this phase. Was my life good? Did I use the opportunities presented to me? How might I have done or seen things differently at the time? What was the purpose of my life? What do I believe about an afterlife? Did I learn to love well? Such introspection may naturally occur at this time, or may have commenced well before the age of eighty years. And it may only be precipitated by a potentially life-altering illness during this time.

Usually throughout the life cycle, we consciously or unconsciously edit the events of our life, trying to extract meaning. We have all made mistakes. We have hurt others and been hurt ourselves. Through our difficulties, we have learned about life and gained wisdom. We now identify on a more profound level what we learned and what is most important. Our chances to make amends are limited. Identifying and acting on final choices can be significant to our life completion. Nonetheless, the ideal is to arrive with a strong sense of gratitude for our one magnificent life.

In reviewing your life, you could create an opportunity to validate your personal story by writing a letter back through time to your younger self. What would you say? How has your wisdom deepened? What strengths have supported you through time? At a woman's retreat that I attended, the facilitator gave instruction to write a letter of this nature back to our younger self. Imagine your own letter by the following example:

Dear Jeanie,

I have been thinking about you this morning, and wanted to write what is on my mind. You may or may not choose to read this. However, since there's a chance that something I say may sound intelligent to you, I'm going to take a run at it anyway.

Although you are quite a demure girl, I know you pretty much know what you want. I realize no one really understands you. I know that you make an effort to comply with expectations of other people, yet constantly try to wiggle out of that "box." Sometimes, you even try to get rid of *the box*, and that creates quite the kerfuffle.

I know how you hate the words, "Trust me," so I will say, "Believe me, if you dare." Life gets better. Sometimes it takes a while—maybe even years, but it will get better. Yes, there are those people who will always be difficult and you may never understand. There will always be those who don't "get" you, and think your ideas and your decisions are all crazy. But really, eventually it won't matter, honey. You will become so confident in yourself, that it simply won't matter anymore what other people think.

You may not understand this right now, but always remember the fact of the matter is that when you are true to yourself, all judgments from others become powerless. This is your life, and no one is responsible but you. It's your show! You will come to realize that the grit and courage you have been known for will gain strength, and always be good to rely on. These are the tools of your heart and soul—like self-confidence, humor, and bravery. Like speaking your truth, taking a stand for what you believe, and trusting yourself. Each is priceless to always carry with you, dear one. It's like having your Dad's tool chest along with you in the old pickup truck when you had that flat tire on the bridge, and needed to keep going.

I know it's hard to imagine being content and happy when there is so much you have been through. However, I can tell you that from here, there *is* peace of heart. You *will* feel joy. I see moments when you feel both—like when you hike through the pastures, saunter along the creek bank, and shout out your voice from the high bluff. Always remember the joy you feel when cuddling with your cat, Mindy, and that sweet dog, Princess. Go ahead and escape from everything by playing the piano with your heart unzipped. Laugh joyfully when you ride that motorcycle with the cute boy from California behind you on those hot summer nights. Treasure these experiences. If you feel these moments of joy and add more every day, you will actually feel happiness growing in your heart.

Just remember, what you put your mind to will happen. That may be good or it may be bad. So take time to imagine what you want that is good. No matter how crazy or impossible it may seem, keep imagining. Then, take steps to move you toward those dreams, okay?

Here's the deal, Jeanie. You won't be able to do this life twice. You won't be able to go back and start all over again. You have what you need to make this a great life. So have fun. Laugh. Cry. Love. Kick ass. Say, "Yes!" Work diligently. Play. Fight for right, if you need to. Break the norm, sister. Take risks. Go ahead and get rid of the box. Above all, trust yourself. You have good judgment. And at the end of every day, ask yourself if you have any regrets. I can truly say from here, you will rarely regret the things you've done. In the end, you will mostly regret the things you haven't done. So do it. Do it all—whatever you imagine. Just remember to be kind. Oh yes, one more thing. Always trust that your life is a beautiful piece of art that some Divine Intelligence—greater than you and I—really cares about.

One day— when you read this again, you will realize you already knew it all. Just promise me one thing. Stick this note away in your white leather jewelry box. It might make more sense after it has become dog-eared and worn, shuffled here and there, and you have to put your glasses on to find it once again amongst your antique lockets and rings.

Your heart companion,
Jean

There are times we may believe we lack the wisdom we most need. Often, later, our choices begin to make sense to us. We may realize that we had the answers all along. Only with hindsight can we see that our fears, worries, and doubts were illusions. We may then wish that we would have taken risks and would have dared to act much sooner.

So as sages review their lives, they will see their incredible evolving resource of wisdom that developed with each unfolding decade. This is the ultimate opportunity for experiencing self-compassion, self-forgiveness, and self-celebration. Furthermore, it is only by acknowledging the lifelong emergence of female wisdom that we can embrace our lives with the greatest degree of honor.

Respecting Our Evolution

Life is a journey in becoming human. Our human journey is initiated at birth; it continues through our childhood and youth, midlife, our mature years, and death itself.[11] It is about coming into our fullness. It calls for our acceptance and integration of diverse parts of ourselves.

When we courageously look into our past decades, recognize the significant events, and mine the wisdom that prevails, we cannot help but see the changes that have occurred through the years. Our values have changed, novel talents have emerged, and we most certainly have learned from our inevitable follies. We are essentially the same in spirit and, yet, very different.

Evolving Values. By reviewing your history, no doubt insights emerge that reveal changing values that brought you to the present moment. Things that were very important throughout previous decades evolved into different values. It is well to consider what values have guided you, to determine what is different now, and what you know now that you didn't know before.

Our values are integral to our personal authenticity. If you were to paint a portrait of your authenticity at your present age, what would the "authentic woman" that is you look like? What values, beliefs, actions, thoughts, and relationships fit now? How can you gain or regain a luminous sense of your inner life radiating and nourishing the outer world? These are questions that will hopefully rouse discernment about your current values and what really matters now.

Emerging Talents. In a review of your life, it is good to salute your talents. Women are co-creative by nature. Many talents were obvious when we were young children, and subsequent experiences prompted new talents to develop. Now, as seasoned sages, we have had many opportunities to identify new and unique talents.

What have you created that you are most proud of? What is your most obvious unique and valuable talent? How can you share your talents with full respect and honor? How have you, or can you, bring your evolving gifts into the world? Answering these questions can help you recognize the value and necessity of imparting your talents in creative ways to enrich the experiences and lives of others.

Embracing Follies. What are our follies? Our actions may have been adventurous, self-incriminating, foolish, stupid, idiotic, or downright life-altering fun. Decisions we made may have been crazy, reckless, outrageous, embarrassing, humiliating, or silly. We may have even taken wildly courageous action steps when others would not. How can we, as women sages, view our past follies? When we get downright honest, name them, and identify how we have viewed them, we then may begin to understand lessons from each experience. And there may be occasions when a little self-forgiveness is necessary to liberate our wisdom. This may be the case with an experience that we wish had not transpired in the way it did. We may have denied wisdom to reveal itself due to shame or guilt that had taken hold of our hearts.

It is wise to remember that cautious, careful people, always casting about to preserve their reputation and social standing, do not bring about effective change. Those who really are in earnest are likely to be willing to do *something*, even if taking action may seem privately, or sometimes publicly, foolish. In avowing appropriate sympathies and support, we may be willing to bear consequences that may just end up as a flaming folly. Nonetheless, the risk may well be worthwhile.

Therefore, approach your follies with gratitude, kindness, and self-compassion. Furthermore, begin to claim all learning and wisdom that emerged from a questionable experience. You can then connect your follies to gems that offer wisdom. How can you impart this wisdom to other women, daughters, children, and grandchildren? How can you encourage others that all experiences in life matter and can muster positive results in the long run? Remember, follies are the basis of great and entertaining teaching stories that are likely not to be forgotten!

Exalting Our Female Wisdom

There is a paradox that accompanies aging. Interior awareness often becomes richer while physical abilities slowly lessen. However, it is life-giving to honor and affirm our female wisdom and the intelligence of our bodies, even as we experience our decline. Although it is important to consciously honor body intelligence at any age, this becomes more crucial as we approach our eighties and nineties. Undeniably, it is from our bodies that our Sagessence illuminates.

When physical changes occur, we can deny them, or we can attend to the wisdom held in our bodies. We can listen with keen ears to its messages, and take prudent action, or inaction, accordingly. Accepting that our sensual capacity becomes a source to enliven connections to life, we can access remarkable inspiration. We can also look to the seasons of nature for understanding and integrating the truth of our oneness with all creation. Indeed, there is a mysterious intelligence that resides in our bodies. We become more deeply acquainted with this intelligence through bodily knowing, our bodily expressions and bodily rhythms.

Bodily Knowing. Bodily knowing is a path to wisdom, although the mind has long been regarded as the most reliable source of knowledge and truth. The truth is that your body holds amazing wisdom and has a tenacious memory capacity to guide you through your human experience. As you age, the incredible resource of your body wisdom becomes more apparent. It is essential to attend to and explore the depths of such knowledge.

Bodily knowing may also come in the form of womanly intuition. We have the inherent ability to connect with our inner self, or "higher self." It is a universal, intelligent life force that exists within us all. It is a *knowing* without *knowing why* you know. It is a natural ability in all of us to know everything we need to know.

Intuition may also be subconscious, prophetic, or instinctive. We may become aware through a feeling or an emotion, gooseflesh, or a sign or symbol. It could be a flash of inspiration or an "aha!" moment. Intuition may come in the way of a recurring thought, dream, or a nagging hunger to pursue an idea or take action. Nonetheless, the intuitive heart seems to have access to an infinite supply of this type of intelligence, even information that we have not gathered directly through personal experience.

Bodily Expressions. Deepening sensuality is another path to wisdom. Women's capacity to experience intimacy, sexuality, and sensuality are not limited by age. Limited thinking that considers sensuality as only applying to our intimate relationships is partial and inadequate. Expansive thinking includes depths of bodily expression to include other aspects of life. Take a moment and image bodily expressions through dance, playing a musical instrument, listening to music, reciting poetry, walking in the woods, or even swimming. Examples are boundless.

Whether single, divorced, widowed, or married, women continue to care deeply about the expression and integration of these aspects of bodily expression. These expressions are sources of passion, creativity, spontaneity, and female wisdom. Denial means not simply the loss of a segment of our reality, but the loss of our possible connections with life.

Bodily Rhythms. Awareness that your body is sacred and wise will lead to a new experience of aging. This provides a third path to female wisdom. It is one that precipitates fresh perspectives on the rhythms of life that are integral to your lifelong experience as a woman. It prompts a deeper understanding of your body that has always been integral to your nature. It is tied to the rhythms of all creation.

Connecting our own cycles as women to those of the Earth is a path to female wisdom, and fundamental to our sense and honor of divinity. From the beginning of time, the Universe's creativity emerges from collapse and chaos to reformation; nothing is lost. Constellations change and are woven into others. This is also true for women and provides assurance of ongoing creative transformation inherent in all rhythms of life. This awareness is reassuring in our aging as we continue to experience seasons of life, intrinsic to all of nature—including humanity.

Revering Our Sagessence

Revering our *Sagessence* emerges from our liberating heart work. Our commitment to living our Sagessence is for our own fulfillment, for our families, our communities, and for future generations. As sages, we truly understand that we are on a Divine assignment. Recognizing the depth of our individual unique wisdom, we call upon our resources to facilitate change for greater emotional, spiritual, and social development. Significant change comes from within our own sage heart and mind as we remain willing and open to our evolving development. As we dare respond to a calling of the sage, let us trust the emergence of our sacred metamorphosis, as reflected in the following poem from *Fire in the Well*:

The Sage Comes

After years and years,
finally . . .
the wise sage comes.

With compassionate acceptance
your sage welcomes everything back—
all you wished would be different,
old wounds, scars, and limps,
lost innocence, possessions, loves,
wildness you and others tried to tame,

dreams that remained formless,
fears that attempted conquest,
humiliation that nearly crippled,
grief leaving remnants of quiet anger,
confusion that disturbed your path,
relationships that eroded with time.

Time is what the inner sage says
is needed to finally understand
that all mattered, all was necessary,
for a deep artful texture and
rich, transfixing, colorful grain
of your true divine magnificence
to emerge from the one and only
truly jaded shadow—
that is the horrific misperception
that you should have been perfect,
or whatever should be different.
No, not even so.

After years and years,
finally . . .
you will hear your sage speak.

Everything brought you to now.
Now, hold each morsel of your life
with tenderness,
honor as gems—
otherwise, wisdom is shamed,
unique creations are dishonored,
authenticity risks being aborted.
And, with tender self-compassion,

open to the great embrace
that allows immersion
into true love—you loving you,
that the gods gifted as only yours.

The sage says, this we do lest
we succumb to the madness
of severing ourselves from peace.
Thus, we must thank the wounds,
the scars, and the limps.
Choose forgiveness and love,
set free wildness that seeks
to ride dreams into new realities,
live passionately, confidently,
bid farewell to all that trusts not
the absolute beauty of our lives.
Then, graciously bow to wisdom—

That bequeaths the sage's call.[12]

As we imagine awakening fire in the heart of the sage, various issues of aging are considered—from challenging cultural views to creating liberating images, practices, and lifestyles of aging. In reframing our own process, we establish a new foundation to positively transform views and practices that have been personally limiting. Although this new territory has not been fully developed, we are wise to draw upon the wisdom of experience as well as exploring new visions ongoing.

Imagine your aging as a sacred spiral that provides a dynamic infrastructure for living a richer and more gratifying evolution to finish your life well. Such an image provides opportunities to effect the change that reflects the true nature of a panentheistic Universe, and *that* is core to the soul of woman. We are co-creators with God. Therefore, we can co-create anew elements of hope and fulfillment for later decades as women living our *Sagessence*.

Living Sagacity-in-Action

The second half of life is the time to unveil completely the wonder of you, and fully embrace who you have become. With a wise heart, acknowledge the benefits of your aging. Come to view aging as an important and rewarding developmental stage of life in which you will become more of who you truly are. Your bravery will be obvious to others. Living authentically is the only way you can live. You will be better skilled than at any other life stage to continue mastering psychological, relational, emotional, social, and spiritual development.

We can enthusiastically consider all the possibilities before us as we live longer lives than previous generations. With joyful anticipation, Gay Gaer Luce stated, "I am dazzled by the possibility of living out all the hidden facets of my personality: my unused talents, my suppressed yearnings to see the world, my desire to offer service, my wish to test my strengths and fears and talents, my search for knowledge and love."[13] Yes, possibilities are endless. To imagine that we would be "dazzled" by all that could become a reality during our lifetime is an awesome outlook.

Living into an emerging sage archetype, we live in radically different ways than previous generations lived. We model wisdom consciously and intentionally to inspire positive differences for this and future generations. Our focus is on inner qualities of aging, rather than external qualities imposed by our culture. In sharing our talents and intelligence, we keep seeking answers about what difference we make, or can make, and for whom we make a difference. No doubt, answers to these questions precipitate purposeful, sensible motivation in committing to our dreams and contributions for the world.

As women sages, we create innovative traditions, weave new values, and experience greater continuity of generations. These contributions to the interdependence of all age groups will generate vital results. We see the importance of emerging family narratives and stories of human relationships, and their continuance with historical depth. A vital gift to succeeding generations is our documentation of our ancestral history, our own lives, and the happenings of our current generation.

Utmost is our responsibility to bring dynamics of woman sage leadership into our emerging legacy. We imagine transcendence utilizing core values of trust, love, acceptance, gentleness, joy, generosity, patience, and hope. We commit to continued action necessary to create such a cultural and global shift.

Lastly, as women sages, we embody the faith and courage required to surmount prior expectations of aging. Our strength conveys more certainty as we find intuitive ways to share gifts of wisdom. The stand we take now will not be forgotten, as we comprehend that the leadership of each woman sage matters to the health of the whole world and its continuing evolution.

Begin to envision your own new images of evolving leadership. As you dare to ponder the magnitude of your place in the immense universe in which we dwell, may awe and wonder begin to prevail in your heart. If you imagine viewing the movement of the planets from an inclusive vantage point in the sky and witness their relationship one to another, you may begin to grasp that your existence in the scheme is nothing less than miraculous. According to astronomers' best estimates, there are at least one-hundred billion galaxies in the observable universe. You participate in this system as well!

Our small phase of time in this existence is precious. Our opportunities to leave our footprints are vast. The time is *now* to celebrate life. Michael Learner eloquently reminds us,

> We know that we will soon be dead and another generation will come after us to look up at this same sky, experience the same awe. *But this is our moment.* Surrounded by those whom we love, we join in song and dance to celebrate the many joys of being alive.[14]

When we come to the awesome realization that this *is* our moment, we can celebrate the liberating journey of our aging. Let us enthusiastically tend to the fires in our hearts urging us to bring about a new global legacy. May we live into content exhaustion as pioneers of this new frontier. As we awaken to the fact that we can claim the name of "sage" in our own right and in our own time, we can also be confident in our own unique wise sage leadership in whatever ways we envision. If we can *dream* of making a transformational difference in our culture at this moment in Universe time, why not *live* it?

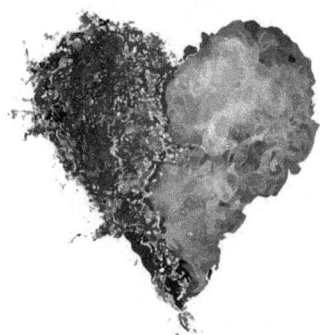

Epilogue

Awakening Fire in the Heart

♥

Amongst all of the "miracle moments" that I have experienced in my life, I count the time I picked up one specific brochure at a conference as one of the most life-altering. A year later, in October 2002, I was cleaning my home office focused on creating order from disarray that had accumulated. There was junk mail, marketing materials, and massive pieces of expired information. As I sat on the floor, I tossed numerous pieces of paper into heaps of those things that no longer mattered. There was little that I deemed valuable.

My attention was suddenly captured and drawn to a brochure I acquired the year prior at the Association of Global New Thought Conference in Palm Springs. The brochure described the Doctor of Ministry Degree program at the University of Creation Spirituality (UCS) in Oakland, California. About ten years prior and during what I call my "spiritual renaissance," I had studied the book *Creation Spirituality* by Matthew Fox, as well as many other books by this spiritual master. His teachings were pivotal in the process of re-envisioning my own spirituality. The UCS brochure relative to Creation Spirituality had caught my eye, as nature had always been my most beloved sanctuary.

As I read the brochure that day, I sensed that the information had come to my attention again at a perfect moment in time. After I read every word, I sat upright on the floor of my office. The message was clear; I must start planning to attend this program. There was not a question whether to take the next step—just a question of when. I decided to apply for admission to the university.

The following year, I attended my first class with the intention of completing a Doctorate of Ministry degree. At that time, I could not imagine how this opportunity for personal transformation and spiritual growth would evoke change in my life. I did believe it would provide insights to change the focus of my work and my way of being in the world. As I reflect on my career including areas of audiology and psychology, I clearly see the foundation for an evolution toward the birth of a vocation through learning gained at that university—which has since evolved into Ubiquity University in San Francisco.

During my career, I have had the privilege of working with individuals who experience hearing loss. In my private audiology practice, the primary population of patients was senior citizens. The journey to success with patients, from diagnosis to rehabilitation of hearing loss, is generally fraught with many negative issues. Typically, primary challenges come with assisting the person to move through stages of grief relative to their sensory deficit. Many individuals require support in helping them acknowledge their essential responsibility in facilitating successful communication with their loved ones, friends, and colleagues. Occasionally, a person may have gone through the aural rehabilitation process without achieving what I considered initial critical steps. In such a case, there

♥

was usually a negative perception about their hearing loss relative to aging that lingered with that person and hindered progress.

There are longstanding cultural beliefs that when one is hearing impaired, they are considered disabled and/or old. This perception is underscored with the general negative view of aging in our country. It generates added resistance in moving forward with rehabilitation, although strong cultural demands for precise and accurate communication prevail. Individuals who are influenced by negative cultural perceptions of aging often sacrifice hearing rehabilitation even though it could support a more fulfilling and joy-filled life. In averting hearing rehabilitation, they also succumb to the incredible health risks resulting from lack of brain stimulation that involve memory challenges, dementia, and Alzheimer's disease.

My experiences with people over the age of fifty expanded as I concurrently worked in the field of psychology. I saw older women courageously working through life-altering situations, and facing challenges of how to live productive and fulfilling lives in their later decades. I became increasingly aware of the need to shift cultural views of becoming older. In examining psychological blocks to embrace the aging process, the prevailing ideology of youth could not be overlooked. Furthermore, I believed it was essential to scrutinize the bell curve paradigm of life that our society has endorsed.

As I investigated my own personal inquiries and deepened my knowledge relative to aging, I developed more creative, compassionate, and diverse approaches to working with individuals. I began seeing my senior patients as women and men who carry an abundance of wisdom that continues to multiply throughout the years. Although each person has exclusive wisdom, many do not feel qualified to share their truth. These "seniors" are not just projects for physicians, audiologists, counselors, families, and friends. Each deserves to be treated with the utmost respect, dignity, and honor. I began to see opportunities to challenge society's limiting model of aging simply by how I chose to encounter others with respect and regard every day.

At the time of completing requirements for my doctorate, I was leading women's classes, retreats, and seminars relative to aging issues. The concept of *Sagessence* emerged. Subsequently, there came the necessity to develop a business model that is Sagessence, LLC. The ministry of Sagessence, LLC is to promote affirmative transformation of personal and cultural views that honor aging. Our goal is to support women and men in honoring their life stories, in claiming their unique life wisdom, and in developing creative strategies to manifest a dynamic life. We believe that by creating liberating images of aging, honoring affirmative change, and consciously living as sage leaders, we can more fully contribute to our families, communities, and future generations. Thereby, each woman and man activates wholeness in the world.

I believe that personal fulfillment can deepen as we awaken and become more intentional in embracing what is named as the Four Fires of Sagessence. As each of us consciously re-envisions our sacred life path, it is wise to awaken to the Divine presence everywhere and especially relative to our aging. Our potential for a vital, fulfilling life during this time increases as we open to new visions. A radical change in cultural views of aging requires stirring newness in our hearts and minds regarding ways of living. We then can create informed choices to manifest transformation in our lives.

My work in the world now continues to evolve from a fire of personal desire to contribute in the development of charting a contemporary path for women sage leaders to be exemplary in their aging. I believe women will be instrumental in fostering exponential change that is deeply needed. It will involve discernment of our work as sages, and movement toward ideals of women in sage leadership. Such leadership is envisioned to be dynamically greater and more fulfilling than our present ideals of living in the second half of life. This is necessary for our personal health, the health of society, our environment, and the world.

We can be certain that everything is at stake at this time and in this century as we move toward cultural transformation. New visions and contributions in the second half of life, individually and in the community, will greatly affect our future. As we embrace opportunities with openness in preparation for unexpected possibilities, it is important to realize that the power to change the world lies in our ability to align our thoughts and actions for evolved, mature outcomes. We must resist whatever pulls us back into the familiar past. When a vision is alive in the mind and we open ourselves for the neoteric wizardry to emerge, we also prepare for the work that will be necessary to facilitate its mission.

So one may wonder what it is that prevents true change. My simple answer, or not so simple answer, is our feelings and our emotions. Feelings and emotions are the end products of an experience. When we are in the midst of any experience, our five senses are gathering sensory data.

Information is immediately sent back to the brain through our five sensory pathways. As this occurs, neurons organize themselves to reflect that event. The moment these nerve cells become patterned into networks, they fire into place and release chemicals. Released chemicals create emotions. In other words, emotions and feelings can be viewed as neurochemical memories of past events.

If emotions imprint experiences into long-term memory, we will most likely talk ourselves out of our ideas when we are faced with obstacles that require new ways of thinking and behaving. We will reject a possibility for change when we use familiar feelings as a barometer for change. Since our feelings reflect the past, they are familiar to us in the sense that they have already been experienced. To live into change requires us to shift or sometimes abandon past ways of thinking, acting, and feeling so we can move into the future with new outcomes. This requires us to take courage in fostering conversion, and claim our masterful authorship in creating the life we desire.

Transformation requires us to alter and expand our thinking and behavior beyond familiar feelings that root us in past behaviors and attitudes. If we succumb to familiar feelings of fear, worry, frustration, sadness, greed, or self-importance in the midst of transformation, we will surely abort change. Most likely, we will return to our old feelings, emotions, and perceptions of self, sinking back into performing old familiar behaviors.

How can we then begin to approach shifts in our lives? First, hope for change requires us to think independently from cultural views. Then we begin by examining our own emotions, feelings, and perceptions. When we develop the skills to do so, we will then facilitate physiological changes in the brain, the mind, and the body to prepare us for the future.

We need to cultivate our art of self-reflection to identify behaviors that limit change. The art of self-reflection is dying in a technological culture saturating us with so much information that many people become addicted to the external world as they rely on outer conditions to stimulate their thinking. As sages, we must carve out solitude to quiet our minds in order to envision ourselves in new ways. We meditate apart from external world stimuli; we plan our futures and mentally rehearse the behaviors we want to change. We ponder new ways of being. As we awaken the fire in our hearts, we will surely set ourselves apart from a typical societal destiny.

Although my focus here has been to rouse fire in the hearts of women specifically, let me be clear that I believe men are also called to serve as sage leaders at this time in history when a sage archetype is emerging. We are the manifestation of a new vision of *great way showers* in the world. As we embark on the Four Fires of Sagessence, we will indeed set ourselves apart from the norm. Most importantly, we will contribute to the Divine's endless birthing of good in the world. We have the opportunity to live the most meaningful lives ever lived on Earth. We are called to keep faith in our new visions. As sage leaders consciously living our Sagessence and integrating the Fires of Authenticity, Passion, Compassion, and Vision, we will create opportunities for greater personal fulfillment and influence meaningful changes for the greater good in this generation and future generations.

In closing, I invite you to take a few moments to reflect on a poem I wrote in response to the posed question,

"How has my life mattered?" Take a moment to consider further, "How can my life really matter from here?" You may even question whether you can absolutely claim the name of *sage* wholeheartedly with all that has happened in your life—yes, considering *all* that has happened. Let me reassure you, beautiful one, that all of your life has mattered. All situations, circumstances, victories, and losses are the threads that created the amazing tapestry that has woven the beautiful art that is your life.

Believe in the wisdom of your years. Tend to the fires in your heart. Know that your time is now for the liberating journey as a sage. Come to your life celebrating the exquisite intelligence that is you!

Come to Your Life

Regardless of what you think
your life should have been,
or what you have believed
could have been better choices,
or what voices said to tempt
your heart to turn and run;
regardless of what you know,
what you don't know, or
what you wish to understand—

Come to your life today
with an open, healed heart,
allow your dear soul
to reflect its deeper truth,
increase your capacity to love,
emulate your unique wisdom.

Epilogue

♥

Simply come . . .
with greater appreciation
for all that has been before.

Come to your life filled,
not empty.
Wrap your arms around you.
Kneel to the mysterious calls
you hear from the gods.
Arrive at your place shouting
to the Universe to prepare
for your living an even more
exquisite version of you.[1]

As you accept the name of sage, stay true to your authentic voice. Believe in the wisdom of your years. Continue to offer your gifts with love. You will be known as a sage with vision. Perhaps your next generation will look back on your time and honor the cultural transformation that you courageously bridged, and they will celebrate the liberating journey of their own aging.

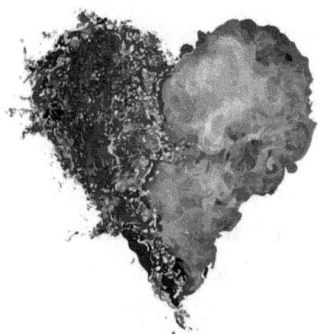

Appendix

Ceremony and Celebration

♥

Ceremonies mark significant events in our lives. They are particularly important for women sage leaders as they birth the image and accept their responsibilities. A ceremony is typically a set of actions that has symbolic importance for the people performing it. It metaphorically refers to a pattern that functions as a connection. An important function of ceremony is to highlight and affirm the continuity of certain valued aspects of relationships.

Another function of ceremony is to mark changes in relationships. We traditionally symbolize these important changes with ceremonies such as graduations, weddings, baptisms, and funerals. Constructing formal ceremonies can symbolize important changes of relationship, both of people with each other and of people with themselves.

There are virtually no formal ceremonies or informal celebrations that center on the acknowledgement of wisdom or initiation for sages in our Western culture. It is valuable for us, as women to create ceremony, ritual, and celebration around claiming our wise spirits and the emergence of our Sagessence. Activities in this regard not only create meaning and significant opportunities to mark the embodiment of the sage in celebration, but also create a legacy for future generations.

As we acknowledge our need for ceremony and celebration, we provide a context in which to recognize and reflect on important events or changes in our lives, including the process of aging. It also provides support from a community of women, while allowing that community an opportunity to adjust its perceptions of the initiation calling, and the perceptions of other participants. In other words, ceremony and celebration facilitate alternative perceptions of women's aging. As we create ceremony, it is well to ask what experience or context would change women's perceptions of their aging and/or evidence of aging challenges. If we do not take opportunities to create ceremony and celebrate the arrival of the sage, women may have difficulty making transitions into conscious sage leadership.

As women co-create ceremonies, there are two basic strategies. First, we imagine the structure with a clear intention for the ceremony. We can modify the format, shape the dynamic flow of the process, and remain open to its ongoing development. Second, we can deepen our experience of ceremony by applying the wisdom we continue to gain. By nurturing and shaping the process of creating ceremony, it will continue to evolve into a container for more meaningful potential.

In the process of developing a ceremony, initial questions may be, "What do I envision that I, or other women, will discover in partaking in this ceremony?" "What might I have not known if I were not participating in it?" These questions invite us to imagine ourselves participating in a ceremony while intentionally remaining open to discoveries that may emerge while participating. What is truly important is the learning we gain through ceremony and celebration. Of further importance is understanding the power of embodiment, which is an essential component of a well-developed and integrated ceremony. By means of embodiment, we carry forth the experience of the ceremony. These suggestions imply that in opening to the rich depth of our imaginations, we can continue to create opportunities for ceremony and celebration beyond the initial experience.

Once we have performed a ceremony in our imagination, it feels more natural to concretize it in the real world. When a woman actively participates in ceremony, the activity then begins to stand for something greater in and of itself. It serves as a rite of passage into a fuller and more rewarding way of living.

Following a ceremony, the next step would then be to reflect on what the ceremony meant to us. What wisdom has the sage gained? How has the sage embodied the intention and experience of the ceremony? The best outcome of a ceremonial experience involves extending meaning into our lives and positively influencing those whose lives we continue to touch.

The element of celebration is essential to any ceremony. Re-envisioning and reframing women's sacred journeys of aging through ceremony include celebratory acknowledgement. At the conclusion of a ceremony, it is a natural sequence to move into the utmost of human experiences: our joyful expressions.

The following *Sagessence Blessing Ceremony* is offered to honor all women sage leaders. Preferably, this ceremony will become a sacred circle ceremony, including ritual and celebration. However, it can easily be modified and performed as a woman's private ceremony.

Sagessence Blessing Ceremony

❤

In preparation for the ceremony, women participants are invited to come together for the common purpose of initiating their sage leadership; and to acknowledge by ceremony and celebration their commitment to live consciously their Sagessence. Prior to the ceremony, women have been instructed to arrive in attire that would individually reflect their conscious choice and desire for initiation and celebration. They have brought with them a touchstone, talisman, or other meaningful object that they have found, purchased, or discovered, that represents to them the abundance of wisdom they have gained throughout their life. Lastly, they have brought their written Initiation Self-Blessing, relative to the emergence of their wise spirits and blessing of the sage.

An altar or center of focus is prepared on the floor in the center of a circle of chairs. A center candle representing "Sagessence" is placed, with four candles that have been chosen to represent the "Four Fires of Sagessence": the *Fire of Authenticity*, the *Fire of Passion*, the *Fire of Compassion*, and the *Fire of Vision*. The candles are placed at four points around the center candle. Other objects can be chosen by the sage leader of the ceremony and could be anything from rocks, shells, containers of water, flowers, or jewelry, to other meaningful objects. Selected music is played softly prior to beginning the ceremony. Written ceremony programs are available for each participant. When time has come to begin the ceremony, drumming or chiming may be chosen to gather attention and direct the women to chairs in the circle.

Welcome

Leader: The leader gives a brief welcome to the group. All the women are then asked to stand and gather into a close circle around the lit candles to participate in the Welcoming Sage Dance (music with appropriate beat and rhythm has been selected). Instructions are given for the circle dance:

1. Place right arm over left arm.
2. Take hold of the left hand of the participant on the left, and right hand of the participant on the right.
3. With left foot, step into the circle one step, and then close with right foot.
4. With left foot, step back outward one step, and close with right foot.
5. With left foot, slide left one step, and close with the right foot.
6. Repeat this pattern throughout the song.

The leader explains the dance as a metaphor: envisioning that as participants step into the circle, they awaken fire in the heart; as they step back outward, they are filled with flames of wisdom; and as they step to the left, they ignite their gifts in the world. Participants are asked to return to their seats at the end of the music.

Introduction

Leader: "As women sages, we come from the Universe that joins all generations. We honor life that moves through time. We honor the stream that flows through us, through our mothers' and fathers' lives, through our grandparents and great grandparents, and by the legacy of all generations past. We acknowledge with reverence the great sacred thread that connects us to our generations—from generations before our birth; and the great sacred thread that flows from us into the generations of our future: our daughters, sons, grandchildren, and generations yet to be birthed. We open our hearts to ignite a sense of Divine interconnection.

"As women sages, we are grateful for the wisdom of the women who have lived before us and honor their names (allow time for participants to name ancestors and those whose remembrance is significant). Their lives have provided a legacy that we can call upon. We accept their legacy of wisdom with reverence. We honor that which passes from generation to generation as sacred."

Incantation

Leader: "As a woman sage, each of you is invited to come to this circle with an intention to embrace the wisdom that has come from your years of living and to acknowledge the empowerment of this gift of wisdom in your life. Open your heart to the Divine's transforming energy of love and generosity, as you welcome your sacred journey of aging.

Come, embrace your wise spirit, welcome the emergence of your sage, and prepare to take responsibility in living your Sagessence as a woman sage leader."

Remembrance

Participants in unison: "With great courage, I have engaged in examining my life—gathering, separating, letting go, grieving, accepting, and celebrating. I have chosen what to take with me into the next phase of my life. I now face myself more honestly than ever before. It is as if I, from this moment, am more integrated and whole than at any other moment before now. I now consciously awaken fire in my heart that reflects wisdom from past generations and from my own life experiences. I am willing to ignite love and devotion to live a legacy for the good of this generation and the next."

Commitment

Participants in unison: "I accept the Divine invitation to tend to:

My *Fire of Authenticity*, a fire that
ignites my genuine truth,
expands my unique creative potential,
nurtures my imagination to birth ideas and dreams,
and inspires liberating images for my life.

My *Fire of Passion*, a fire that
invites me to live passionately in the moment,
to foster love, joy, wonder, and gratitude,
to deepen pleasures in my living,
and to make vital life-affirming choices.

My *Fire of Compassion*, a fire that
stirs me to practice loving kindness,
to live in the flow of loss, grief, and change,
to graciously give and receive care,
and to move through life transitions confidently.

My *Fire of Vision*, a fire that
calls me to create a living legacy that supports greater good,
to manifest deeper fulfillment,
to impart a wise, mentoring spirit,
and to honor intergenerational connectedness."

Initiation with Self-Blessing

Leader: Participants are invited to stand and gather into a circle around the candles. Surrounded by the circle of women, one woman is invited to step into the center and read her self-blessing. Then, remaining in the center, she selects another woman in the circle to read the self-blessing back to her. The second reader then remains in the circle and repeats the process. The blessing ritual continues until the circle is complete.

Wisdom Blessing

Leader: "With the words of Makeda, Queen of Sheba, receive this blessing:

Wisdom is sweeter than honey,
Brings more joy than wine,
Illumines more than the sun,
Is more precious than jewels.
She causes the ears to hear and the heart to comprehend.
I love her like a mother
And she embraces me as her own child.
I will follow her footsteps and she will not cast me away."[2]

Sagessence Blessing

Participants in unison recite the following blessing:

"In celebration of my *Sagessence*,

I honor my personal authenticity.

I bless my day visions and night dreams, and claim my *wise spirit* to forge new paths when necessary.

I bless my forehead, and claim my *wise spirit* of reason.

I bless my eyes, and claim my *wise spirit* of vision to see clearly the beauty of all living things.

I bless my lips, and claim my *wise spirit* to speak the truth about my experiences.

I bless my heart and claim my *wise spirit* to deepen my self-love and in so doing deepen my love for others.

I bless my hands, and claim my *wise spirit* as an artisan for a new humanity.

I bless my womb, and claim my *wise spirit* in co-creating with Divinity.

I bless my feet, and claim my *wise spirit* in continuing to walk my unique path, while honoring the paths of courageous foremothers and sisters.

In blessing my life, I contribute to wisdom legacies of women before me.

And, as I live into my feminine fullness, I will continue to celebrate living my *wise spirit.*"

Vision of Transformation

Participants recite, one voice at a time for each statement, continuing around the circle:

"I will challenge my personal and societal views of older women, and identify ways to embrace new visions.

♥

I will tend to my inner life, and continue to explore new and varied elements of discernment.

I will be mindful and sensitive in the process for continuing change during my life passages, and embrace transitions while honoring my endings and beginnings.

I will continue imparting a wise mentoring spirit, and live my spiritual legacy for the good of future generations.

I will practice new ways of deepening my wisdom, and create new opportunities to connect with others.

I will embrace my value of bodily knowing, and continue to increase my capacity for awareness.

I will open myself to learning from my losses and follies, and live with a sense of compassion, gratitude, and forgiveness.

I will become a catalyst for healing adverse cultural views that have divided us, one from another.

I will envision that all sages will be spiritually, emotionally, and relationally rich in their aging.

I will also hold the vision that all women will celebrate with a spirit of liberation as their years unfold.

And, my prayer is to live in harmony as a *way shower* for others to live harmoniously with each other and with our Earth."

Honoring Women's Wisdom

Leader: The sage leader hands a small candle to each participant. Each woman is invited to share her touchstone, talisman, or other meaningful object, and an explanation of it as a metaphor or remembrance of her abundance of sage wisdom.

A shawl is placed around the shoulders of the first woman to speak. She lights her candle from the Sagessence candle in the middle of the circle and holds the candle while sharing her remembrance. She then places her candle near the Sagessence candle on the altar. As she returns to her seat, she removes the shawl and places the shawl around the shoulders of the woman to her left. Sharing continues until the circle is complete. (Optional drumming can be incorporated between voiced sharing.)

Proclamation

Leader: "May you impart a wise mentoring spirit, be a living example of personal authenticity, and make a conscious commitment to a compassionate, vital life-affirming second half of life. May the beauty of your fullness as a woman shine forth as you live as a sage leader from the center of your wisdom gained from living the sacred journey of your life!"

Closing

Participants: Women gather into a close circle around the candles, to close with the Welcoming Sage Dance (music and dance steps are previously described in Welcome above). At the conclusion of the dance, each woman is invited to take her candle from the circle of candles, and hold it high above her head, taking a few moments to visually acknowledge each woman around the circle.

Leader: "Go and let the fire in your heart burn, and the light of your sage shine forth in the world."

Celebration

An informal celebration follows. Opportunities are given for participants to continue celebrating informally with food, drink, and conversation. Sage leaders are encouraged to offer toasts in celebration.

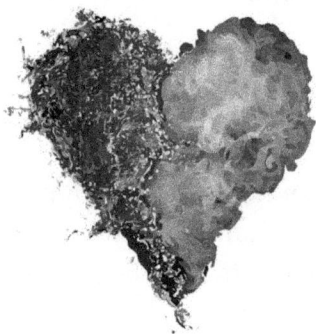

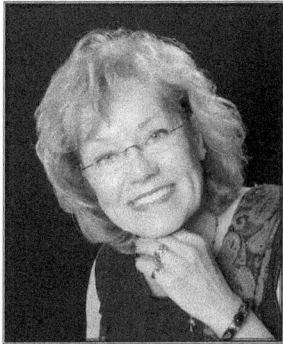

About the Author

💜

Dr. Marilyn Loy Every holds a Doctor of Ministry in Wisdom Studies, with a focus on aging, and certification in Spiritual Direction from Ubiquity University, San Francisco, California. She also holds a Master of Arts in Counseling Psychology from St. Martin's College in Olympia, Washington, a Master of Science in Audiology from the University of Wyoming, and a Bachelor of Science from the University of Nebraska. She specializes in aging issues, communication strategies, life transitions, loss and grief, and spiritual companioning with individuals and in sacred circle groups. She has spent nearly thirty years working extensively with individuals fifty years and older. Marilyn lives in the beautiful Pacific Northwest, United States, where nature is her sanctuary and family is her inspiration.

As a visionary, Dr. Loy Every's passion involves challenging the previously socially accepted paradigm of aging, and supporting the potential emergence of a new life-affirming paradigm. While Western culture has historically idealized youth and early life, it is essentially devoid of respected positions of elders, crones, sages, and wise women and men. Dr. Loy Every believes that re-envisioning aging is essential and foundational to completing our lives with a deeper sense of purpose and meaningful fulfillment. Furthermore, in learning new possibilities in aging, embracing liberating images and honoring change, we can more fully share with, and contribute to our families, local and global communities, and create positive change and transformation for the greater good of future generations.

Dr. Loy Every is founder of Sagessence, LLC, a company with a mission to develop and facilitate programs that inspire women and men to re-envision aging in the second half of their lives. Current classes, programs, seminars, presentations, and keynotes are available through Sagessence, LLC, and include:

- Aging with Purpose, Passion, and Fulfillment
- Sage Leadership Training
- Affirmative Aging Guidance
- Life Visioning for the Second Half of Life
- Women, Wisdom, and the Power of Aging
- Creativity and Wisdom
- Seven Gems of Wisdom Intelligence
- Living Our Sagessence
- Sacred Poetry as a Way of Life

Dr. Loy Every offers the program "Sacred Poetry as a Way of Life" as a corresponding program to her book, *Fire in the Well—Poetry for Women Awakening the Inner Sage.* This poetry book is a companion to *Women and the Liberating Journey of Aging—Awakening fire in the heart.*

Dr. Alexandra Kovats, Spiritual Director and Professor of Spirituality at Seattle University, acclaims:

Dr. Loy Every's poems invite women to explore their sacred journey of aging with grace. They encourage the expression of a woman's authentic wisdom voice. Her soul-scape is imprinted by the powerful beauty of nature, as she calls us to fierce bodily knowing, fiery courage, and naked heartedness. Reading her poems is a sensual feast, and provides true nourishment for the soul.

Visit the Sagessence website at www.sagessence.com

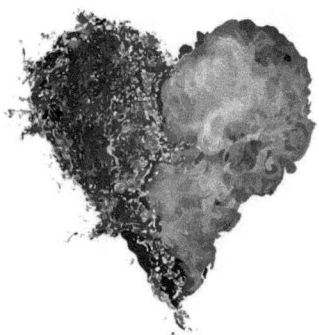

Reference Notes

♥

Epigraph

1. Loy Every, Marilyn. *Fire in the Well: Poetry for Women Awakening the Inner Sage*. Canada: Influence Publishing, 2014, 151-152.

Chapter 1: The Sage Coming of Age

1. Fischer Kathleen. *Autumn Gospel*. Mahway, NJ: Paulist Press, 1995, 20.
2. Costello, R. B., et. al. (Ed.), *Webster's College Dictionary*. New York: Random House, 1991, 323.
3. Fischer, Kathleen. *Autumn Gospel*. Mahway, NJ: Paulist Press, 1995, 7.
4. Sadler, William. *The Third Age*. Cambridge, MA: Perseus Books, 2000, 2-4.
5. Fischer, Kathleen. *Autumn Gospel*. Mahway, NJ: Paulist Press, 1995, 1.
6. Sadler, William. *The Third Age*. Cambridge, MA: Perseus Books, 2000, 11.
7. Ray, Paul and Sherry Anderson. *The Cultural Creatives*. New York: Three Rivers Press, 2000, 8, 12-13.
8. Field Belenky, Mary, Blythe McVicker Clinchy, Nancy Rule Goldberger, and Jill Mattuck Tarule. *Women's Ways of Knowing*. New York: HarperCollins Publishers, 1997, 15.

9. Brooks, Jane. *Midlife Orphan*. New York, NY: The Berkley Publishing Group, 1999, 20.
10. Tolle, Eckhart. *A New Earth*. New York: Penguin Group, 2005, 97.
11. Jay, M. *Sage Leaders and Sage Leadership*. wordnet. princeton.edu/pcrl/webwn, 2008.
12. Ray, Paul and Sherry Anderson. *The Cultural Creatives*. New York: Three Rivers Press, 2000, 295.
13. Loy Every, Marilyn. *Fire in the Well: Poetry for Women Awakening the Inner Sage*. Canada: Influence Publishing, 2014, 6-7.
14. Fox, Matthew. *Passion for Creation*. Rochester, VT: Inner Traditions, 2000, 129.

Chapter 2: The Fire of Authenticity

1. Osho. *intimacy: Trusting Oneself and the Other*. New York, NY, St. Martin's Press, 2001, 30.
2. Fox, Matthew. *Illuminations of Hildegard of Bingen, text by Hildegard of Bingen with commentary by Matthew Fox*. Santa Fe, NM: Bear, 1985, 30.
3. Tenneson, Joyce. *Wise Women*. New York: Bulfinch Press, 2004, 50.
4. Fischer, Kathleen. *Autumn Gospel*. Mahway, NJ: Paulist Press, 1995, 11.
5. Loy Every, Marilyn. *Fire in the Well: Poetry for Women Awakening the Inner Sage*. Canada: Influence Publishing, 2014, 25.
6. Sheehy, Gail. *Sex and the Seasoned Woman*. New York: Random House, 2006, 11-12.

7. Borysenko, Joan. *A Woman's Book of Life*. New York: Riverhead Books, 1996, 240.

8. Tenneson, Joyce. *Wise Women*. New York: Bulfinch Press, 2004, 57.

9. Sheehy, Gail. *Sex and the Seasoned Woman*. New York: Random House, 2006, 297-298.

10. Munro, Alice. *Hateship, Friendship, Courtship, Loveship, Marriage*. New York: Vintage Books, 2001, 323.

11. Schulte, Christa. *Tantric Sex for Women*. Alameda, CA: Hunter House Publishers, 2005, 8.

12. Carrellas, Barbara. *Urban Tantra*. Berkeley, CA: Celestial Arts, 2007, 7.

13. Fischer, Kathleen. *Winter Grace*. Nashville, TN: Upper Room Books, 1998, 12-14.

14. Johnson, Elizabeth. *She Who Is*. New York: The Crossroads Publishing Company, 1995, 135.

15. Loy Every, Marilyn. *Fire in the Well: Poetry for Women Awakening the Inner Sage*. Canada: Influence Publishing, 2014, 90-91.

16. Nicholson, Shirley. *The Goddess Re-awakening*. Wheaton, IL: The Theosophical Publishing House, 1989, 108.

17. Artress, Lauren. *The Sacred Path Companion*. New York: The Berkley Publishing Group, 2006, 11.

18. Loy Every, Marilyn. *"Granddaughter's Lullaby."* Unpublished music composition, 2007.

19. Artress, Lauren. *The Sacred Path Companion*. New York: The Berkley Publishing Group, 2006, 11-12.

20. Fischer, Kathleen. *Autumn Gospel*. Mahway, NJ: Paulist Press, 1995, 71.

21. Williamson, Marianne. *Imagine*. United States of America: Rodale, 2000, 39.
22. Fitzgerald, Kathleen. *Soaring Spirits*. Moon Township, PA: GlaxoSmithKline, np.

Chapter 3: The Fire of Passion

1. Fox, Matthew. *Meditations with Meister Eckhart*. Rochester, VT: Bear & Company, 1983, 93.
2. Follmi, Danielle and Olivier. *Offerings*. New York, NY: Stewart, Tabori & Chang, 2003, January 13-14.
3. McGowen, Kathleen. *The Source of Miracles*. New York, NY: Fireside, 2009, 176-178.
4. Loy Every, Marilyn. *Fire in the Well: Poetry for Women Awakening the Inner Sage*. Canada: Influence Publishing, 2014, 72-73.
5. Oriah. *The Invitation*. New York: HarperCollins Publishers, 1995, 12.
6. Loy Every, Marilyn. *Fire in the Well: Poetry for Women Awakening the Inner Sage*. Canada: Influence Publishing, 2014, 55-57.
7. Fox, Matthew. *Creation Spirituality: Liberating Gifts for the Peoples of the Earth*. San Francisco: Harper, 1991, 19.
8. Fox, Matthew. *Creation Spirituality: Liberating Gifts for the Peoples of the Earth*. San Francisco: Harper, 1991, 19.
9. Jackson Gandy, Debrena. *All the Joy You Can Stand*. New York: Three Rivers Press, 2000, 19-20.
10. Shinoda Bolen, Jean. *Crones Don't Whine*. York Beach, ME: Conari Press, 2003, 82-83.

11. Meister Eckhart as quoted in Fox, Matthew. *Passion for Creation*. Rochester, VT: Inner Traditions, 2000, 81.

12. Loy Every, Marilyn. *Fire in the Well: Poetry for Women Awakening the Inner Sage*. Canada: Influence Publishing, 2014, 61-62.

13. Jackson Gandy, Debrena. *All the Joy You Can Stand*. New York: Three Rivers Press, 2000, 230.

14. Byrne, Rhonda. *The Magic*. New York, NY: Atria Books, 2012, 16.

15. Fischer, Kathleen. *Autumn Gospel*. Mahway, NJ: Paulist Press, 1995, 93-94.

16. Loy Every, Marilyn. *Journal Entry*. Unpublished Journal, 2004.

17. Peeke, Pamela. *Body for Life for Women*. United States of America: Rodale, 2005, 17-18.

18. Roundtree, Cathleen. *On Women Turning 50*. New York: HarperCollins Publishers, 1993, 113.

19. Loy Every, Marilyn. *Journal Entry*. Unpublished Journal, 2006.

Chapter 4: The Fire of Compassion

1. Fox, Matthew. *A Spirituality Named Compassion*. San Francisco: Harper, 1979, 30.

2. Fox, Matthew. *The Coming of the Cosmic Christ*. New York: HarperCollins Publishers, 1988, 32.

3. Kornfield, Jack. *The Wise Heart*. New York, NY: Bantam Dell, 2008, 23.

4. Williamson, Marianne. *Imagine*. United States of America: Rodale, 218.

5. Williamson, Marianne. *Imagine*. United States of America: Rodale, 245-254.

6. Fox, Matthew. *Passion for Creation*. Rochester, VT: Inner Traditions, 2000, 170, 213-225.

7. Loy Every, Marilyn. *Fire in the Well: Poetry for Women Awakening the Inner Sage*. Canada: Influence Publishing, 2014, 89.

8. Fischer, Kathleen. *Winter Grace*. Nashville, TN: Upper Room Books, 1998, 144-146.

9. Foster, Lavina. *"Memories."* Unpublished poem, 1982.

10. Loy Every, Marilyn. *Fire in the Well: Poetry for Women Awakening the Inner Sage*. Canada: Influence Publishing, 2014, 87-88.

11. Morrow Lindbergh, Anne. *A Gift from the Sea*. New York: Pantheon Books, 1975, 24-25.

12. Loy Every, Marilyn. *A Day to Let Go*. Unpublished poem, 2010.

13. Loy Every, Marilyn. *Fire in the Well: Poetry for Women Awakening the Inner Sage*. Canada: Influence Publishing, 2014, 85-86.

14. Loy Every, Marilyn. *Fire in the Well: Poetry for Women Awakening the Inner Sage*. Canada: Influence Publishing, 2014, 106-107.

15. Loy Every, Marilyn. *Fire in the Well: Poetry for Women Awakening the Inner Sage*. Canada: Influence Publishing, 2014, 83.

Reference Notes

♥

Chapter 5: The Fire of Vision

1. Loy Every, Marilyn. *Fire in the Well: Poetry for Women Awakening the Inner Sage.* Canada: Influence Publishing, 2014, 132-133.
2. Mazer, Gwen and Christine Alicino. *Wise Talk, Wild Women.* San Francisco: Council Oak Books, 2007, 73.
3. Wheatley, Margaret. *Turning to One Another.* San Francisco: Berrett-Koehler Publishers, 2002, Epitaph.
4. Shinoda Bolen, Jean. *Crones Don't Whine.* York Beach, ME: Conari Press, 2003, 107-113.
5. Ellison, Sheila. *If Women Ruled the World.* San Francisco: Inner Ocean Publishing, 2004, 63-64.
6. Barks, Coleman. *The Soul of Rumi: A New Collection of Ecstatic Poems.* New York: HarperCollins Publishers, 2001, 79.
7. Schaefer, Carol. *Grandmothers Counsel the World.* Boston: Trumpeter, 2006, 118.
8. Ellison, Sheila. *If Women Ruled the World.* San Francisco: Inner Ocean Publishing, 2004, 13.
9. HH Dalai Lama and Howard C. Cutler. *The Art of Happiness.* New York: Riverhead Books, 1998, 293-315.
10. Williamson, Marianne. *Imagine.* United States of America: Rodale, 2000, 11-16.
11. Harris, T. "The question of a lifetime: What will you do with the gift of an additional 14 years?" *Spirituality & Health,* 2000 Winter 2(4), 22-25.
12. Corey, Gerald. *Theory and Practice of Counseling and Psychotherapy.* Pacific Grove, CA: Brooks/Cole Publishing Company, 1996, 168, 170-180.

13. Corey, Gerald. *Theory and Practice of Counseling and Psychotherapy*. Pacific Grove, CA: Brooks/Cole Publishing Company, 1996, 97-102.

14. Makeda, Queen of Sheba as quoted in Hirshfield, Jane. *Women in Praise of the Sacred*. New York: HarperCollins Publishers, 1994, 14.

15. Loy Every, Marilyn. *Fire in the Well: Poetry for Women Awakening the Inner Sage*. Canada: Influence Publishing, 2014, 117-118.

16. McAdams, D. *Generativity: The New Definition of Success*. Spirituality & Health, 2001 Fall, 4(3), 26-33.

17. Fischer, Kathleen. *Autumn Gospel*. Mahway, NJ: Paulist Press, 1995, 15.

18. Reilly, Patricia. *A God Who Looks Like Me*. New York: Random House, 1995, 102.

19. Loy Every, Marilyn. *Fire in the Well: Poetry for Women Awakening the Inner Sage*. Canada: Influence Publishing, 2014, 121-123.

20. Radmacher-Hershey, M. "*Living Eulogy*." Printed poster, 1997.

Chapter 6: Tending Fire in the Heart

1. Van Eyk McCain, Marian. *Elderwoman*. Scotland: Findhorn Press, 2002, 179.

2. Borysenko, Joan. *A Woman's Book of Life*. New York: Riverhead Books, 1996, 33.

3. Borysenko, Joan. *A Woman's Book of Life*. New York: Riverhead Books, 1996, 58.

4. Borysenko, Joan. *A Woman's Book of Life*. New York: Riverhead Books, 1996, 117.

5. Borysenko, Joan. *A Woman's Book of Life*. New York: Riverhead Books, 1996, 143.

6. Borysenko, Joan. *A Woman's Book of Life*. New York: Riverhead Books, 1996, 148.

7. Borysenko, Joan. *A Woman's Book of Life*. New York: Riverhead Books, 1996, 150.

8. Borysenko, Joan. *A Woman's Book of Life*. New York: Riverhead Books, 1996, 190.

9. Borysenko, Joan. *A Woman's Book of Life*. New York: Riverhead Books, 1996, 223.

10. Loy Every, Marilyn. *"Aging."* Unpublished poem, 2015.

11. Brennan, Anne and Janice Brewi. *Passion for Life*. New York: The Continnum Publishing Company, 1999, 30.

12. Loy Every, Marilyn. *Fire in the Well: Poetry for Women Awakening the Inner Sage* Canada: Influence Publishing, 2014, 148-150.

13. Williamson, Marianne. *Imagine*. United States of America: Rodale, 2000, 255.

14. Williamson, Marianne. *Imagine*. United States of America: Rodale, 2000, 271.

Epilogue

1. Loy Every, Marilyn. *Fire in the Well: Poetry for Women Awakening the Inner Sage*. Canada: Influence Publishing, 10.

Appendix

1. Loy Every, Marilyn. "*Sagessence Blessing Ceremony*." Unpublished ceremony.
2. Makeda, Queen of Sheba as quoted in Hirshfield, Jane. *Women in Praise of the Sacred*. New York: HarperCollins Publishers, 1994, 13.

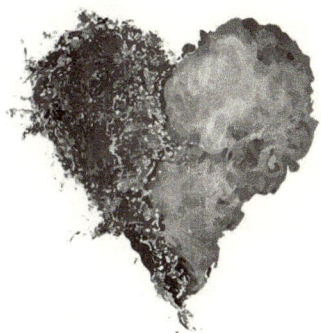

www.ingramcontent.com/pod-product-compliance
Lightning Source LLC
Chambersburg PA
CBHW031426270326
41930CB00007B/595